# Francine Prince's VITAMIN DIET for Quick and Easy WEIGHT LOSS

WITH A FOREWORD BY
BERNARD MELTZER
Leading Consumer Advocate

CORNERSTONE LIBRARY
Published by Simon & Schuster
New York

**Caution:** This book is not intended by the author or publisher as medical advice, and is not to be regarded by the purchaser as such. Any such advice, particularly as it pertains to diet and exercise, should be obtained from your physician. The author and publisher specifically disclaim any liability, loss, or risk, personal or otherwise, resulting as a consequence, directly or indirectly, from the use and application of any of the contents of this book.

Copyright © 1982 by Francine Prince
All rights reserved
including the right of reproduction
in whole or in part in any form
Published by Cornerstone Library
A Simon & Schuster Division of
Gulf & Western Corporation
Simon & Schuster Building
1230 Avenue of the Americas
New York, New York 10020

CORNERSTONE LIBRARY and colophon are
trademarks of Simon & Schuster, registered in
the U.S. Patent and Trademark Office.

Manufactured in the United States of America

1   3   5   7   9   10   8   6   4   2

Library of Congress Cataloging in Publication Data

Prince, Francine.
Francine Prince's Vitamin diet for quick and easy
weight loss.

Includes index.
1: Reducing diets.   2. Vitamins—Physiological effect.
I. Title.   II. Title: Vitamin diet for quick and easy
weight loss.
RM222.2.P724          613.2'5          81-19504
                                       AACR2
ISBN 0-346-12521-9

*To today's dieters
who will be tomorrow's
slim
and healthy people*

# Contents

PART III
MAKING THIS DIET WORK *FOR YOU*
—MORE RAPIDLY AND HEALTHFULLY

# Foreword

Over the last fifteen years more than 100,000 people from all over the nation have called in to my radio show and said, in essence, "Dr. Meltzer, I have a problem. I need help." I pride myself that in a few minutes the anxiety is gone from each caller's voice, and a happy person says, "Thank you."

These days when a caller's problem concerns dieting, nutrition, or cooking for better health, I almost always answer with words of wisdom from Francine Prince's books. Her advice is down-to-earth and grows out of life experience. She realizes it's more important to know how to shop in the supermarket for slimming, healthful food that's priced right, and to be able to prepare that food deliciously, than it is to parrot a lot of medical generalities that have little or no application in our day-to-day lives. She speaks my language and yours.

I became an ardent fan of Francine Prince's philosophy of "practical nutrition" after reading her first three best sellers, *The Dieter's Gourmet Cookbook*, *Diet for Life*, and *Francine Prince's New Gourmet Recipes for Dieters*. A lot of diet books, as you may well know from your own sad experience, don't deserve to be best sellers, but Francine Prince's books certainly do. She asks the question, "Can diet help bring about a slimmer, fuller, healthier, and longer life?" and answers with a resounding "Yes!" with eloquence and good humor, and all the facts you need to make her practical nutrition work for you.

Since finding a diet that can help you become more attractive and lead a more productive and zestful life is of interest to almost everyone, I invited Francine Prince for a guest appearance on my radio program, "What's Your Problem?" The audience loved her! She received more than 4,000 letters—a record—and for months afterward people kept calling to ask when she would be back on the show. She says she'll have the time to make more guest appearances after this book is published. Keep tuned!

Which brings me to *this* book: *Francine Prince's Vitamin Diet for Quick and Easy Weight Loss*. I think it is her most important book. It's about time the nation had a reducing diet that's healthful not harmful, that's delicious not dull. Her Vitamin Diet is sound and safe because it's based on Dr. Norman Jolliffe's Prudent Diet, which has been acclaimed by doctors everywhere as the best and most healthful diet ever created. What Francine Prince has done is to update and upgrade Dr. Jolliffe's famous diet and make it taste like four-star restaurant fare.

The Vitamin Diet works because it's so practical. This is no carrot stick and celery

11

diet; you can eat *real* food, the kind of food you're used to—and lots of it. You can stay on this diet in restaurants as well as at home. You don't have to cook a single dish if you don't want to; but if you want to, you can follow her recipes in her *Vitamin Diet Mini-Cookbook*, which is a bonus book within this book. And let me tell you, if you've never tasted a Francine Prince recipe before, you're in for a treat. Also, this diet *insists* you snack four times a day—and any dieter will tell you, *that* is the height of practicality.

But what I like most about the Vitamin Diet is it doesn't let you down once you reach your ideal weight. You go right on eating all the approved foods you want, and eating all the approved vitamins, and you stay slim for the rest of your life. If you've tried other diets and are as fat now as you were before, or even fatter than you were, try *this* diet. It's simple to follow, easy to stay on, and delicious to eat.

If you were to call me on my radio program and say, "Dr. Meltzer, I have a problem. There are so many diets. Which one should I go on?" I'd say, "If your doctor says the choice is yours, go on Francine Prince's Vitamin Diet. It's really not a diet at all. It's a wonderful new way to eat for the rest of your life for the sake of your life—slimfully and healthfully."

Bernard Meltzer
NBC Radio Network Consumer Advocate
Host "What's Your Problem?"
WOR Radio, New York

# PART I

## Why This Diet Is Like No Diet You've Ever Been On or Heard of Before

# 1

# THE DIET THAT SUCCEEDS WHEN EVERYTHING ELSE FAILS

I didn't just write this book—I lived it.

I'm slim, zestful, vigorous proof that the diet you'll find in it *works*.

*It works* because you can shed unsightly excess weight encouragingly fast—up to ten pounds, sometimes more, of even the most stubborn water and blubber in just one week.

*It works* because you can stay attractively slim for the rest of your life automatically—with no effort on your part.

*It works* because you eat until you're full—at three complete meals and four satisfying snacktimes a day.

*It works* because you can stay on this diet in most restaurants—there's no break with familiar eating patterns, no disruption of your lifestyle.

*It works* because you don't have to cook a single meal—but if you do decide to cook, the recipes are indescribably delicious.

*It works* because, although calories do count, you don't have to count calories—it's all done for you.

*It works* because it has none of the unpleasant side effects of fad diets—it's healthful, not harmful.

*It works* because you eat the foods you like—All-American favorites from hamburger to steak, from bread to cake.

*It works* because it controls your appetite *for* you—you'll never binge, chainsnack, or eat compulsively again.

Above all—

*It works because it fulfills every dieter's dream of "magic pills" on which you can reduce and stay reduced.*

The "magic" is the magic of sound scientific principles effectively applied. The "pills" are not pills at all, but the basic foods on which all life depends—vitamins.

## THIS DIET IS BASED ON THE ONLY ONE TESTED IN REAL LIFE BEFORE RELEASE TO THE PUBLIC

The Vitamin Diet is an upgrade of a diet hailed by the medical profession worldwide as "the most phenomenally successful in medical history"—the Prudent Diet, developed by the late Dr. Norman Jolliffe. As director of the Bureau of Nutrition, New York City Department of Health, he persuaded the Commissioner of Health, Dr. Leona Baumgartner, to sponsor a breakthrough nutritional experiment—a test of his diet in real life.

Most diets fail long-term because they're tested under restricted conditions—at fat farms, clinics, hospitals, or under the strict supervision of diet doctors. When released from restrictions, almost all dieters return to their fat eating habits and gain weight. The only way to decide in advance whether a diet would work, Dr. Jolliffe realized, was to test it without restrictions.

"Here's your diet," Dr. Jolliffe instructed his 1,100 volunteers. "Stay on it if you can, but otherwise live the way you always have." "There was no attempt," observed pioneer nutritionist Arthur Blumenfeld, the foremost historian of the Jolliffe experiment, "to induce them to make the slightest change in their way of life."

The dieters, a cross-section of overweight New Yorkers, lived in their own "filled-fridge" homes, ate in their favorite restaurants, went to parties, took vacations, snacked in the movies and before their TV screens—carried on under the same diet-threatening conditions you encounter every day. To Dr. Jolliffe, this was "a public trial" of his diet—a trial *by* the public *for* the public.

And the public won—*big*. The results, Blumenfeld reported, "made front-page news [and] medical history." Almost all of the 1,100 "human guinea pigs" (Dr. Jolliffe used the term affectionately) reduced to their ideal weight. Even more astonishing—at the end of four years, only a few had put back some of the weight they had lost. On other diets, 95 percent of dieters put back within a year *all* the weight they had lost.

"Immediately . . . all over the world . . . the Prudent Diet became medically recognized," Blumenfeld wrote, "as the best type of reducing diet."

Dr. Jolliffe's milestone results were achieved using highly motivated members of his Anti-Coronary Clubs (his "human guinea pigs") who were for the most part not excessively overweight. With more difficult-to-reduce patients at his Obesity Clinics, Jolliffe, according to nutrition authority Jane Brody, claimed "only that most men stayed on the low-fat Prudent Diet for many years. His own estimate of the long-term success of clients attending Obesity Clinics was 30 percent, *still a lot better than other diets*" [emphasis mine].

My diet upgrades the 1952 Jolliffe diet in the following ways: It is more restrictive in the use of fat, saturated fat, and cholesterol; is higher in fiber; contains considerably less sugar (sucrose) and salt; and contributes RDAs of minerals and optimal quantities of vitamins.

The key to the success of this diet, as it was to the success of the Jolliffe diet, is the control of the body's appetite-regulating mechanism, the *appestat*. The appestat is controlled today, as it was three decades ago, by the proper nutritional mix. That mix *now* includes optimal vitamin supplements to compensate for the shortfall of natural vitamins in many of the foods most Americans eat—hence the name, "Vitamin Diet."

The Prudent Diet succeeded when everything else failed. The Vitamin Diet can be called a Super Prudent Diet.

# 2

# YOU CAN SHED UP TO 10 POUNDS, LOOK FANTASTIC, AND FEEL WONDERFUL IN JUST ONE WEEK

I discovered that it can be done—the discovery came as a result of the great success of my previous three bestsellers. I was so much in demand to demonstrate my famous haute cuisine of health that I was often away from home for weeks at a time appearing on major TV and radio shows, at the flagship stores of national health food chains, and at leading book shops and department stores. Eating three meals a day away from the stay-slim larder in my Manhattan kitchen, I couldn't help but gain weight.

After one extended trip, I stepped on my bathroom scale and was horrified to discover I had put on 10 bulging, unbecoming pounds. I had the same "Oh-my-God-what-have-I-done!" feeling you may have had after you returned from that cruise or vacation resort or that long holiday visit with the folks. My predicament may have been worse than yours because I was to appear the following week on a national TV show before about 50 million viewers—and what kind of advertisement would I be for my kind of cuisine, which promises: "Eat like a gourmet—and stay slim forever"?

Oh, I could have taken my excess weight off slowly, one to three pounds a week, while eating my fill of my delectable dishes, but *I had only 7 days to drop 10 pounds.* What was I to do?

Fad diets were out—much too dangerous. I think it's senseless to lose weight with diarrhea, or the threat of uric acid poisoning, or with a symptom of diabetes, or with the menace of pernicious anemia. I didn't want to drag myself around for a week with one or more of the following fad-diet side effects—foul breath, dizziness, weakness, nausea, vomiting, leg cramps, constipation, and vicious hunger pangs. Certainly, with the eye of the TV camera soon to focus on me, I couldn't afford that haggard victim-of-Dracula look I've seen on every fad dieter I've ever known.

I love food—don't you?—and I didn't want to punish myself with days of nothing but mixed fruit (The Beverly Hills Diet); with normally crisp dishes that taste as if they had been doused with a water hose ( the Scarsdale Diet); with rolls made *only*—this is incredible!—with egg yolks, stiffly beaten egg whites, and an artificial sweetener (the Atkins Diet); or with raw vegetables, which I'd have to lug around all day long and nibble on continually (the Pritikin Diet). I'm a nutritional hedonist. I believe that if eating is not an enjoyable experience, no matter what you eat, it's no good for you. I had been accustomed to my own slimming and healthful recipes, called by food critics "a miracle . . .

mouth-watering . . . the food of the Gods"—and I wasn't going to settle for a diet composed of ugh-ly food.

Where could I find a crash diet that would be tasteful as well as healthful?

But even if I could find such a diet, would it be wise to go on it? Losing a good deal of weight in a hurry, some diet experts tell you, can upset your body's delicate chemical balance and bring about all sorts of woes. Even Dr. Richard Stuart, psychological director of Weight Watchers International, the giant take-it-off corporation, warns that rapid weight loss could have deleterious effects on your physical and emotional well-being. Dr. Jean Mayer, the world-renowned nutritionist, advises weight loss of only a pound a week ("That's fifty-two pounds a year," he points out). The evidence seemed so strong against precipitate poundage drops that in my previous books I had recommended a maximum weight loss of only three pounds a week.

Yet I was faced with a problem that only a crash diet could solve. I had to look svelte and gorgeous on that national TV show, and I had only a week in which to do it.

If anybody would have had a solution to my dilemma, I thought, it would have been the late Dr. Jolliffe. I hustled over to a nearby medical library and plunged into an in-depth study of his work—papers in scientific journals, his classic textbook, *Chemical Nutrition*, and his breakthrough diet book, *Reduce and Stay Reduced*—and I found the answer.

Dr. Jolliffe wrote, "There are reports of 10 to 12 pounds of weight lost through water excretion in the first week of the diet. Five to 7 pounds is not uncommon." Although Dr. Jolliffe never used the term "crash diet," a diet on which you can lose 5 to 12 pounds or more in one week *is* a crash diet. I quickly brought it up to date and went on it at once. When the famous TV host exclaimed, "And now meet America's leading authority on cooking for better health—Francine Prince!" I never looked slimmer or felt more energetic and vibrant. I was thrilled by what my new One-Week Crash Diet had done for me.

You'll be as thrilled by what it will do for you.

## YOU CAN START ON THIS DIET THIS MINUTE

Eager to get started? Then don't waste time. Turn to Chapter 7 (page 30), and get going. Then, as you watch the numbers on your bathroom scale go down, down, down, and see a slim new you emerging in your full-length mirror, come back and read *why* this marvelous transformation is happening to you.

*Caution:* This diet is based on the ex-

periences of my husband and myself, and our study of nutritional literature. Before going on this or any other diet, obtain the approval of your physician, preferably a nutrition and/or diet specialist. While you're on this or any other diet, visit your physician for periodic monitoring.

# 3

# FINALLY—A CRASH DIET THAT'S HEALTHFUL, EASY TO STAY ON, AND DELICIOUS

"Fine, it works," people say to me. "But I'm not going on your Crash Diet until you answer some questions."

Sensible. Go ahead.

*Every diet I've ever been on had side effects. What side effects did you experience?*
None. Unless you call having the time of my life a side effect.

*Can a crash diet actually be healthful, not harmful?*
Most doctors would probably answer "No." But I build my "Yes" on the following facts:

• Dr. Jolliffe wrote, "The greater the overweight the faster the weight reduction may be. Within the standards of a satisfactory diet, this is sound practice, for the more overweight the more dangerous it is."

• *Excess* water in the body can lead in some cases to high blood pressure, "the silent killer." When some or all of the excess water is released, blood pressure in those cases could drop toward normality. On this diet, rapid weight loss is achieved by releasing some or all of your excess water.

• Water-soluble vitamins and minerals that may be lost as water is flushed away are replaced by adequate supplements.

• When water is released, water-swollen tissue shrinks, giving you a slimmer look. Puffiness tends to disappear. Just look in the mirror and see what a change water loss can make in your appearance.

• Weight reduction is due to water loss at the outset, then to fat loss. Fat loss during my Crash Diet is accomplished on about 1,200 to 1,600 calories a day, depending on your size (a range recommended by the Bureau of Nutrition, New York City Department of Health). The amount of fat shed is from 2 to 2½ pounds a week, a quantity that is medically accepted as safe and desirable for most dieters.

• The Crash Diet introduces you to a healthful diet which long-range can help ward off heart attack and other degenerative diseases. You'll find that this kind of diet is so palatable—and when you use my recipes, so delicious—that you'll want to stay on a maintenance version of it for the rest of your life for the sake of your life.

19

*You're the leading authority on cooking for better health, so I suppose you expect me to cook, right?*

Wrong! I *don't* expect you to cook. I want to make that point so clearly that I'm putting it into a headline—

# YOU DON'T HAVE TO COOK A SINGLE ITEM

*Does that mean I can eat out while I'm dieting?*

Yes, in most restaurants, including some ethnic ones.

*And can I eat supermarket foods?*

Sure.

*It looks like the easiest crash diet ever. What's the catch?*

No catch. You simply eat the kinds of food you've liked all your adult life. This Crash Diet is so easy to stay on that I once thought of calling it The Supermarket Crash Diet or The Eat-Out Crash Diet.

*I've looked over your Crash Diet menus and I like them. But couldn't I have something special now and then?*

Certainly. That's why I've included here a book within a book—*The Vitamin Diet Gourmet Mini-Cookbook* (pages 99–198). It's packed with a *new* super-delicious haute cuisine of health recipes. Just substitute the appropriate recipes for the dishes on my One-Week Crash Diet Menus. I repeat, you don't have to

cook, but if you use my recipes just a few times a week, you'll turn a wonderful week into an unforgettable one.

*I've never cooked before except making eggs or broiling a steak. Am I going to miss out on your slimming recipes everybody says are so delicious?*

No way. My recipes are so simple to follow that you can get them right the first time even if you've never cooked *anything* before. You can't imagine the joy ahead of you. Cooking my way is exciting, stimulating, creative. It's a form of self-expression like writing, painting, dancing. It makes you feel *so* wonderful! All this—and rapid weight loss, too. No other diet can make this claim.

*I never in my life heard that vitamins can help you reduce and stay reduced. I wish you could give me some scientific proof.*

You'll find that proof—facts that *are* completely new to you—presented in everyday language beginning with the following chapter.

# 4

# THE BREAKTHROUGH DISCOVERY
# BEHIND THIS REVOLUTIONARY
# VITAMIN DIET

Face this eye-opening truth: You're not overweight because you have a glandular imbalance, or because your parents were fat, or because you're unlucky in love. You're overweight because you eat too much.

But you *can* cut down on food over load effortlessly, automatically, and, most important, *naturally*. You'll never again have to resort to potentially dangerous, and often useless, over-the-counter and prescription diet pills.

The secret is learning how to take command of a mechanism, built into your body, that regulates the amount of food you eat. Here is how that mechanism works, as described by its discoverer, Dr. Norman Jolliffe:

"As a thermostat will automatically adjust the furnace so as to keep the temperature of the house constant, so will the *normal* weight-regulating mecha-

nism adjust the appetite . . . and keep the weight constant."

He added, "As a convenient term by which to refer to this mechanism, I have coined a word for it—the *appestat*. The appestat is located in the hypothalamus, [a gland] which is in the brain at the base of the skull."

The appestat sends out an enough's-enough signal—that contented filled-up feeling—when the food you eat brings in just enough calories, minerals, and vitamins to satisfy your body's needs.

But, like a thermostat, your appestat can be set too high. When it is, the enough's-enough signal doesn't go off until you've consumed more food than you need. Then you're fat.

You can help prevent that from happening when you take command of your appestat with the right amount of vitamin supplements.

## HOW VITAMIN SUPPLEMENTS HELP CONTROL YOUR APPETITE FOR FAST, NATURAL, AND PERMANENT WEIGHT LOSS

Your appestat is naturally set at normal. That means you eat food containing the right amount of calories to keep you at ideal weight, and the right amount of

vitamins to keep you at peak health and efficiency. Here's how that situation looks in a diagram:

## FOOD CONSUMED TO KEEP YOU
## AT YOUR IDEAL WEIGHT

Appestat

NORMAL

Calories

Vitamins

But let's say the food you consume supplies the right amount of calories you need, but only half the amount of vitamins.

## FOOD CONSUMED TO KEEP YOU
## AT YOUR IDEAL WEIGHT

Calories

Vitamins

Then the appestat sets at a higher level to bring in twice as much food to supply you with the full amount of vitamins you need.

## FOOD CONSUMED TO KEEP YOU
## AT YOUR IDEAL WEIGHT

Appestat

HIGH

Calories

Vitamins

You're now consuming twice as many calories as you need, and your weight soars.

But if you add the proper amounts of vitamin supplements to your food . . .

### Vitamin Supplements

### Vitamins

. . . the appestat setting returns to normal . . .

## FOOD CONSUMED TO KEEP YOU AT YOUR IDEAL WEIGHT

**Appestat**

NORMAL

**Calories**

**Vitamin Supplements**

**Vitamins**

. . . and you're once more consuming only the amount of calories you need to maintain your ideal weight.

Since you're now consuming far less calories, you'll lose weight—naturally, rapidly. When you reach ideal weight, you'll stay at it—automatically.

The Vitamin Diet supplies the right amount of vitamin supplements. Used this way, vitamins become the "magic pills" for taking it off fast and making it last.

---

*Caution:* The appestat is not immediately reset to normal upon the addition of optimal vitamin supplements to your diet. It takes many weeks. But the appestat level *begins* to lower at once; a lower level means less food consumption, and less food consumption means weight reduction. Other factors besides vitamins influence the level of the appestat (I'll tell you about them as we go along); and *vitamin supplements alone will not induce weight loss.* Weight loss is accomplished only when my entire dietary program is followed.

# 5

# WHY YOU DON'T NEED DIET PILLS, AND WHY YOU DO NEED VITAMIN SUPPLEMENTS

*You call vitamin supplements "magic pills" for taking it off fast and making it last. Are they drugs?*

They are not, even though they're sold where drugs are sold, and come in the tablet, capsule, or drop forms familiar to the drug user. Vitamins are nutrients just like carbohydrates, proteins, fats, and minerals. They are a vital part of the biological processes in every cell of the body. Without vitamins there can be no life. Drugs, on the other hand, even when medically prescribed, are alien invaders that can disrupt the normal biological processes and, when used in overdoses, can produce grim side effects, including death.

Diet pills are drugs, vitamins—the "magic pills"—are foods.

*What's wrong with diet pills? I understand Americans buy billions of dollars' worth of them a year.*

These are the facts:

Diet pills, which can be found in every size, shape, and color in drugstores throughout the country, consist mainly of the following ingredients: PPA (phenylpropanolamine hydrochloride), a nasal decongestant present in cold tablets; benzocaine, a constituent of anesthetic-antiseptic sprays; and caffeine. PPA is claimed to short-circuit the appetite, benzocaine to numb your stomach and discourage your desire to eat, and caffeine to lift your spirits while you're undergoing the diet-pill ordeal.

High blood pressure is the major potential hazard from this trio of drugs. Teresa A. Young of the Federal Drug Administration's Philadelphia office reports that other maladies attributed to diet pills include fainting, cramps, fatigue, and irritability. She says, "We don't recommend any brand names. They don't actually work the way they claim."

*What about amphetamines and dexedrine? They're diet pills with a proven record of success.*

True. They were once the most widely prescribed appetite suppressants. No more. They're addictive.

*I've been told I get all the vitamins I need in my food. Why do I need supplements?*

You do *not* get all the vitamins you need in your food. Jane Brody, the esteemed columnist of *The New York Times*, writes of "vitamin shortfalls in the overly processed American diet." Robert J. Benowicz, a leading authority on vitamins, adds: "Highly respected scientists, medical authorities, and government agencies offer compelling evidence that vitamin concentrations [in our foods] fall far short . . . of levels for maximum good health."

*Why are the foods we eat vitamin-poor?*
Here are some of the reasons:

• Fruit is plucked green, and vegetables are harvested before they're ripe. There's no chance for the full quota of vitamins to develop.
• Virtually all the food we consume goes through processing—a massive chemical and mechanical assault that decimates vitamin content.
• Long-distance shipping and extended storage-life cause vitamins to deteriorate.
• Vitamins are lost in the kitchen by freezing, thawing, peeling, paring, slicing, cooking, and reheating.

Most foods that reach our tables contain only minuscule amounts of their normal vitamin quotas. The vitamin C in a cooked potato has been depleted by 1,000 percent, according to the U.S. Department of Agriculture.

And whatever vitamins you do get in your food are almost completely wiped out by smoking, pollution, alcohol, caffeine (in coffee, tea, Cokes, and drugs), oral contraceptives, prescription and over-the-counter drugs, and stress. Vitamin supplements are necessary not only to help you control your appetite, but also to help keep you healthy and vigorous.

Now I'll ask a couple of questions:
*What day of The One-Week Crash Diet are you on? And how many pounds have you lost?*

If you haven't started yet, turn to Chapter 7—and get going.

# 6

# BREAK YOUR COMPULSIVE EATING HABIT WITHOUT A SINGLE PANG OF HUNGER

If you're like nine out of ten compulsive eaters I've met, you'll say to me, "What—me, a compulsive eater! Ridiculous!"

Really?

Take this test. It's a variation of one originated by Marcia Seligson of *Cosmopolitan* magazine.

Select one of your favorite foods. What is it? Chocolate-chip cookies? Okay. Ask Miss Slim (or Mr. Slim) if she's as fond of chocolate-chip cookies as you are. She *is?* Good!

Now serve a huge bowl of chocolate-chip cookies. Watch Miss Slim as she eats. Does she gobble up every chocolate-chip cookie in sight? No way. She eats only as much as she needs, leaving a mound of goodies untouched.

Do you?

If you don't, you're a compulsive eater.

*I failed the test. Now tell me, why am I a compulsive eater?*

Your appestat is set high. You'll feel compelled to eat and eat and eat until the appestat sends out the enough's-enough signal. And that signal won't come for a long time.

*Then to get rid of my compulsive eating habit, I have to reset my appestat at normal?*

Correct. Dr. Norman Jolliffe wrote, "The appestat . . . this automatic weight-regulating mechanism which operates through appetite [control] is amazingly efficient when normal." Normalizing the appestat is the key to overcoming compulsive eating.

*Then why, even though I'm taking the right amount of vitamin supplements to normalize the appestat, am I still a compulsive eater?*

You're obviously not on my diet. The foods you're eating contain weight-*decontrol* elements that raise the level of your appestat despite the effect of vitamins, weight-*control* elements that lower the level of your appestat. Weight-decontrol elements are sugar, salt, and excess fat.

Sugar is the nation's No. 1 food additive; salt is No. 2. Fat supplies 42 percent of the average American diet; all your body needs is 30 percent. Is it a wonder that we're a nation of overweights?

### What steps must I take to get rid of my compulsive eating habit?

Just one easy step. Stay with the *complete* Vitamin Diet. It will normalize the appestat. Here's why:

• *It minimizes all the weight-decontrol elements.* It contains little sugar, salt, and excess fat.

• *It accentuates all the weight-control elements.* It contains the right vitamin and mineral supplements and is high in fiber. "Shrinking-stomach pains" raise the appestat level, and fiber alleviates them. Fiber is found in fruit, vegetables, and grains.

A normal appestat ends compulsive eating—automatically. Allow at least four to six weeks' eating my slimming way (on my reducing and/or maintenance diets) to normalize the appestat.

### Is removing weight-decontrol elements and accentuating weight-control elements healthful?

This is an exceptionally healthful diet, conforming closely to the nutritional guidelines established recently by the U.S. government. It is also low in saturated fat and cholesterol and contains a full complement of minerals.

### Will breaking my compulsive eating habit give me hunger pangs? I couldn't stand that.

Nothing to worry about. Hunger pangs are caused by an unsatisfied appestat. On my diet you eat all you need to satisfy your normalizing appestat. You'll never feel a pang of hunger.

And here's a plus—

Once your appestat is set at normal, you'll be completely satisfied with the meals and snacks on my maintenance diet. *You'll never again feel the urge to binge.* (But you will be able to go on *controlled* binges, as you'll see later.)

# PART II

## THE SIMPLEST, EASIEST DIET EVER CONCEIVED

# 7

# VITAMINS, THE "MAGIC DIET PILLS"— THE KINDS AND AMOUNTS YOU NEED

Take the right vitamin supplements in the right amounts, and on this diet you'll lose up to 10 pounds, and sometimes more, in just one week.

All you need are three kinds of vitamin products. For the number of "pills" of each, refer to the following chart.

## YOUR SLIMMING DAILY ALLOWANCES (SDAs) OF VITAMINS

| | Number of Vitamin "Pills" | | |
|---|---|---|---|
| YOUR AGE: | 19–35 | 36–50 | 50+ |
| Vitamin C (1,000-mg units) | 1 | 1 | 2 |
| Multiple vitamins (A, 5,000 IUs; D, 400 IUs; E, 30 to 100 IUs) | 1 | 1 | 2 |
| Vitamin B-50 complex | 1 | 2 | 4 |

Go out to your drug store or health food store right now and get them. To make buying easy, just clip out the Purchasing Guide on the facing page, and bring it to the vitamin counter.

## WHEN TO TAKE YOUR SLIMMING DAILY ALLOWANCES (SDAs) OF VITAMINS

Take your vitamins with your other food at any of the three major meals of your day. I prefer to take mine as the last course at breakfast.

Stocked up on your three kinds of vitamin products?
Know how many of each to take?
Great!
Now start using them to reduce to your ideal weight fast—and to make it last.

------------------------------------------------------------

# THE VITAMIN DIET
# VITAMIN PURCHASING GUIDE

## VITAMIN C

Ask for 1,000-milligram tablets of ascorbic acid. If you prefer to avoid acidic foods, ask for calcium or potassium ascorbate. They're nonacidic.

## MULTIPLE VITAMINS

Ask for a multivitamin product matching these figures for fat-soluble vitamins:

| Vitamins | Units |
|----------|-------|
| A | 5,000 IUs |
| D | 400 IUs |
| E | 30 to 100 IUs |

Select a multivitamin product which contains as well U.S. RDAs of all essential minerals. The presence of small quantities of other than fat-soluble vitamins in these products can be helpful.

## B–50 COMPLEX

Almost all balanced B–50 products conform closely to the following contents:

| Vitamins | Units |
|----------|-------|
| $B_1$ | 50 mg |
| $B_2$ | 50 mg |
| $B_3$ | 50 mg |
| $B_6$ | 50 mg |
| $B_{12}$ | 50 mg |
| Biotin | 50 mcg |
| Choline | 50 mg |
| Folic acid | 400 mcg |
| Inositol | 50 mg |
| PABA | 50 mg |
| Pantothenic acid | 50 mg |

------------------------------------------------------------

*Warning:* The SDAs are meant as general guidelines. The amounts of vitamins that are best for you depends on a number of variables other than age—such as, the amount of caffeine, alcohol, and drugs you consume; your body weight and size; your stress level, the conditions of your environment, and your life style. Certainly, the SDAs are not applicable to children or to anybody with a health problem. Before adding SDAs, or any vitamin supplements to your diet, consult with your physician.

# 8

# THE COMPLETE VITAMIN DIET— IT'S AS SIMPLE AS TURNING DOWN A THERMOSTAT

Just as a thermostat controls the amount of fuel flowing into your furnace, so does the appestat control the amount of food going into your body. Losing weight and keeping it off simply means turning down your appestat.

*With as few as three vitamin "pills" a day, the Vitamin Diet turns down the appestat for you.*

Once it's turned down you'll never experience hunger pangs on a healthful low-calorie diet; and you'll stay at your ideal weight for the rest of your life— automatically.

*You'll never have to worry about counting calories again.*

"Many people [with normal appestats] go through life without giving their weight a second thought," explained Dr. Norman Jolliffe, a former director of the National Vitamin Foundation, who discovered the appestat. "If they occasionally eat more on one day or at one meal than is needed . . . because of an insistent hostess or anxious mother . . . or because of some particularly delectable portion of food . . . [then] without thinking about it, they eat less at the next meal or the next day."

The wonderful thing about this diet is: your appestat starts to be turned down the first day. Step on your bathroom scale during the first few days, and be thrilled by your weight loss. "I can't stand those one-pound-a-week diets," a small-town housewife said. "I look at my scale, and I look and I look, and nothing happens. It discourages me, and I give up." This diet *encourages* you.

## THE OVERALL DIET PLAN—THE MOST PRACTICAL EVER

You can put this simple plan into action anywhere, at any time. You can eat in, you can eat out. You can party, visit, snack, and even cheat occasionally. You can, in short, diet and enjoy yourself thoroughly. The practical way is the only way to reduce and stay reduced.

My overall diet plan is as easy to stay on as it is simple to follow. All you do is—

# TAKE FIVE EASY STEPS TO LIFETIME SLIMNESS

STEP 1. Go on a *One-Week Crash Diet*, during which you may choose to eat all the approved foods you desire.

STEP 2. Enjoy a *Controlled Binge Week*, during which you binge every other day, and continue to lose weight.

STEP 3. Return to the *One-Week Crash Diet* if you have to lose more weight.

STEP 4. Continue to alternate a *Controlled Binge Week* with a *One-Week Crash Diet* until you've slimmed down to ideal weight.

STEP 5. Stay at your ideal weight automatically with my *Thin-for-Life Program*.

If you need to lose 10 pounds or less, you may only have to take Steps 1 and 5.

# INSTRUCTIONS FOR GETTING THE MOST OUT OF THE VITAMIN DIET

*Warning*: Follow these instructions, and all other instructions in this book, to the letter. Do not improvise, alter, or deviate in any way. During the first weeks, your newly lowered appestat is unstable, and any violation of my instructions could be disastrous. "The appestat," Dr. Jolliffe wrote, "will . . . slip back to its original high level, and then you will overeat and gain fat again." (For exceptions to this warning, see the first question on page 73.)

1. *Decide on your weight goal.* How many pounds do you want to lose? Five, 10, or more? You can do it. But I recommend you set your ideal weight as your goal. That's the weight at which, life insurance statisticians tell you, you're likely to be healthiest and live longest. It's also the weight at which you'll look most attractive.

Find your ideal weight on the following page. Weights are given without clothes for people over 25. If you're between 18 and 25, find your ideal weight for your height, then subtract one pound for each year under 25.

I can't emphasize too strongly that you should set your goal through a consultation with your physician, and report to him (her) periodically while you're dieting. It is those dieters who have tried to lose enormous amounts of weight too fast on fad diets who have suffered untoward side effects—ones that should have been caught through periodic physician monitoring.

2. *Weigh yourself naked before breakfast.* If you don't have a bathroom scale, get one immediately. For the rest of your life, you're going to weigh yourself every morning before breakfast. You will weigh yourself *only* at that time, and *only* on your bathroom scale. Do not move your scale to any other part of your home.

3. *Keep a record in your head of your daily weight loss.* No need for an elaborate scoreboard. You won't forget these figures. Not *these* figures.

4. *Go on the One-Week Crash Diet*

# CHART OF IDEAL WEIGHTS

| Height (feet and inches) | Men Build | | | Women Build | | |
|---|---|---|---|---|---|---|
| | LIGHT | MEDIUM | HEAVY | LIGHT | MEDIUM | HEAVY |
| 4–10 | 95 | 100 | 105 | 90 | 94 | 98 |
| 4–11 | 97 | 103 | 108 | 93 | 98 | 102 |
| 5–0 | 100 | 106 | 111 | 95 | 100 | 105 |
| 5–1 | 105 | 111 | 117 | 97 | 102 | 108 |
| 5–2 | 110 | 117 | 123 | 100 | 106 | 111 |
| 5–3 | 115 | 122 | 128 | 105 | 112 | 118 |
| 5–4 | 120 | 127 | 133 | 110 | 116 | 123 |
| 5–5 | 125 | 132 | 138 | 112 | 119 | 126 |
| 5–6 | 130 | 137 | 143 | 117 | 124 | 130 |
| 5–7 | 133 | 141 | 148 | 120 | 127 | 134 |
| 5–8 | 137 | 145 | 153 | 125 | 132 | 139 |
| 5–9 | 143 | 151 | 159 | 130 | 137 | 144 |
| 5–10 | 148 | 156 | 164 | 135 | 142 | 149 |
| 5–11 | 152 | 160 | 168 | 140 | 147 | 154 |
| 6–0 | 155 | 163 | 171 | 144 | 151 | 158 |
| 6–1 | 163 | 171 | 179 | | | |
| 6–2 | 167 | 175 | 183 | | | |
| 6–3 | 170 | 179 | 188 | | | |
| 6–4 | 172 | 181 | 195 | | | |
| 6–5 | 178 | 188 | 198 | | | |
| 6–6 | 185 | 195 | 206 | | | |

*tomorrow morning.* That's *tomorrow.* Not next week. Not next month. Tomorrow. Remember, there's a sexy, cheerful, radiant, energetic you buried under all those excess pounds. If you want the real you to emerge, start on this safe, healthful Crash Diet *tomorrow.* You'll find the tasty menus in the next chapter.

And one final word to all of you before you plunge into one of the most exciting weeks of your life—

*Dieters of the world, throw away your salt shakers. You have nothing to lose but your weight.*

Good eating, good health, and happy dieting!

# THE ONE-WEEK CRASH DIET: YOU EAT ALL THE APPROVED FOODS YOU WANT

Here are the menus for the next seven days—seven days that could turn your life around.

"But I can't do it without snacks," a young mother at a suburban shopping mall said. "I'd just die if I couldn't snack. Can I snack on your diet?"

## YES, YOU CAN SNACK

The Vitamin Diet is above all a practical diet. It takes all your eating needs into account. To most dieters the most urgent of these is the the need to snack.

On this diet you can snack.

With my guilt-free snacks—

## YOU'LL NEVER BE TEMPTED TO CHAIN-SNACK AGAIN

Here's why:

The snacks that helped put excess weight on you are heavy in appetite stimulants that raise the appestat. A raised appestat causes chain snacking. My guilt-free snacks are free from these stimulants—sugar, salt, and excess fat.

# MY GUILT-FREE SNACKS HELP YOU *STAY* ON YOUR DIET

If you've ever dieted before, you're familiar with the most powerful of all appetite stimulants—"shrinking-stomach pains." They occur between meals, send the appestat sky-high, and send you scurrying for the nearest snacks.

But that won't happen any more. My guilt-free snacks contain a built-in preventive for "shrinking-stomach pains." It's natural fiber—what Grandma used to call "roughage." It balloons in the stomach and gives you the feeling that your stomach hasn't shrunk at all. "Shrinking-stomach pains" never occur, the appestat remains reset, and you stay on your diet.

## THE MOST SATISFYING OF ALL DIETS

On the Vitamin Diet, you can enjoy four snacktimes a day in addition to three regular meals.

You'll eat as much as you desire of such mouth-watering favorites as roast beef, chicken, hamburger, sirloin steak, turkey, fish and other seafood, fruits, grains, and salads.

To lovers of food like us, the Vitamin Diet is the most satisfying of all diets.

Prove it to yourself, starting with the first day's menu, as you shed your excess weight swiftly, simply, safely, and surely.

*Note:* For a discussion of portion sizes see page 73.

# MENUS FOR THE ONE-WEEK CRASH DIET

You can enjoy these in most restaurants, as well as in your own home. Do not cook with or add salt, sugar, butter, cream, or whole milk to any dish. Eat your salad before your entrée. Eat slowly. For super-taste sensations, use recipes from *The Vitamin Diet Gourmet Mini-Cookbook*; it starts on page 99.

# Good news! You have only ⑦ days to go before you binge!

## FIRST DAY

### BREAKFAST

½ grapefruit sprinkled with teaspoon toasted bran or wheat germ, and teaspoon raisins
½ cup spoon-sized shredded wheat
½ cup low-fat milk
Coffee or tea
Your Vitamin SDAs (see chart page 30)

### MID-MORNING SNACK

Guilt-free snacks and beverages (see page 47)

### LUNCH

Salad of watercress, mushrooms and grated carrot
Oil and vinegar dressing (2 teaspoons oil, 4 teaspoons vinegar)
Cold steamed or boiled shrimp with lemon juice
Small apple
Mint tea or club soda with lime

### MID-AFTERNOON SNACK

Guilt-free snacks and beverages

### DINNER

Clear Bouillon (salt-free)
Small broiled hamburger
Sliced onions
Steamed or boiled asparagus and cauliflower
Fresh fruit
Mint tea or club soda with lime

### TV SNACKTIME

Guilt-free snacks and beverages

### BEDTIME SNACK

Cup low-fat milk or plain low-fat yogurt

*Good news! You have only ⑥ days to go before you binge!*

## SECOND DAY

### BREAKFAST

½ cup orange juice
1 scrambled egg made with teaspoon unsalted corn oil margarine, pinch of
   tarragon and 3 dashes ground red
   (cayenne) pepper
1 slice whole wheat toast
Coffee or tea
Your vitamin SDAs

### MID-MORNING SNACK

Guilt-free snacks and beverages

### LUNCH

Salad of lettuce, tomatoes, cucumbers
   and radishes
Oil and vinegar dressing (see first day
   LUNCH)
Steamed cod, sole, or snapper with
   lemon juice
Piece thin-sliced whole wheat bread or
   whole grain wafer
Mint tea or club soda with lime

### MID-AFTERNOON SNACK

Guilt-free snacks and beverages

### DINNER

Sliced tomatoes with lettuce and watercress
Broiled chicken (without skin)
Half-cup each steamed or boiled eggplant and turnip
½ cup canned pineapple chunks in its
   own juices, or fresh pineapple chunks
Mint tea or club soda with lime

### TV SNACKTIME

Guilt-free snacks and beverages

### BEDTIME SNACK

Cup low-fat milk or plain low-fat yogurt

*Good news! You have only ⑤ days to go before you binge!*

## THIRD DAY

### BREAKFAST

Cup of melon balls
Small blueberry or bran muffin
Low-fat cottage cheese (no salt added)
½ cup low-fat milk
Coffee or tea
Your vitamin SDAs

### MID-MORNING SNACK

Guilt-free snacks and beverages

### LUNCH

Salad of shredded zucchini, carrots, and
    sliced pepper
Oil and vinegar dressing (see first day
    LUNCH)
Small broiled hamburger without bun
Whole grain wafer
Mint tea or club soda with lime

### MID-AFTERNOON SNACK

Guilt-free snacks and beverages

### DINNER

Shredded cabbage and carrot salad
Broiled fillet of sole or snapper
½ cup each steamed or boiled broccoli,
    carrots and green beans
½ cup unsweetened applesauce
Mint tea or club soda with lime

### TV SNACKTIME

Guilt-free snacks and beverages

### BEDTIME SNACK

Cup low-fat milk or plain low-fat yogurt

*Good news! You have only 4 days to go before you binge!*

# FOURTH DAY

## BREAKFAST

Broiled grapefruit sweetened with pineapple juice and several dashes ground
coriander
½ cup cooked hot cereal of your choice
(not instant)
½ cup low-fat milk
Coffee or tea
Your vitamin SDAs

## MID-MORNING SNACK

Guilt-free snacks and beverages

## LUNCH

Salad of cucumbers, watercress, carrots
and radishes
Oil and vinegar dressing (see first day
LUNCH)
Open-faced turkey or chicken breast
sandwich
Mint tea or club soda with lime

## MID-AFTERNOON SNACK

Guilt-free snacks and beverages

## DINNER

Tomato juice (no salt added)
Watercress and cucumbers
Broiled baby lamb chop
Small baked potato
½ cup cooked spinach
Fresh fruit
Mint tea or club soda with lime

## TV SNACKTIME

Guilt-free snacks and beverages

## BEDTIME SNACK

Cup low-fat milk or plain low-fat yogurt

*Good news! You have only ③ days to go before you binge!*

## FIFTH DAY

**BREAKFAST**

Cup of tomato juice (no salt added)
Poached egg on slice of whole wheat
   toast
½ cup low-fat milk
Coffee or tea
Your vitamin SDAs

**MID-MORNING SNACK**

Guilt-free snacks and beverages

**LUNCH**

Salad of sprouts, watercress and carrots
Oil and vinegar dressing (see first day
   LUNCH)
Small can of tuna fish packed in water
   (no salt added) with lemon juice (use
   salad dressing with tuna fish rather
   than with salad, if you prefer)
Whole grain wafer
Mint tea or club soda with lime

**MID-AFTERNOON SNACK**

Guilt-free snacks and beverages

**DINNER**

Fresh fruit cup
Broiled chicken (without skin)
½ small baked sweet potato (eat the
   skin, too; save other half)
½ cup green beans or broccoli
Fresh fruit
Mint tea or club soda with lime

**TV SNACKTIME**

Guilt-free snacks and beverages

**BEDTIME SNACK**

Cup low-fat milk or plain low-fat yogurt

# Good news! You have only ☐2 days to go before you binge!

## SIXTH DAY

### BREAKFAST

Whole orange
Cup puffed rice (no salt or sugar added), sprinkled with 2 teaspoons toasted bran or wheat germ
½ cup low-fat milk
Coffee or tea
Your vitamin SDAs

### MID-MORNING SNACK

Guilt-free snacks and beverages

### LUNCH

Mixed green salad with sprouts
½ cup low-fat cottage cheese (no salt added)
Oil and vinegar dressing (see first day LUNCH)
1 slice whole wheat bread
Mint tea or club soda with lime

### MID-AFTERNOON SNACK

Guilt-free snacks and beverages

### DINNER

Chicken broth (salt-free)
Salad of chicory, endive, and cold sweet potato from last night's dinner
Small minute steak
½ cup steamed or boiled green beans
½ cup pineapple chunks in its own juices, or fresh pineapple chunks
Mint tea or club soda with lime

### TV SNACKTIME

Guilt-free snacks and beverages

### BEDTIME SNACK

Cup low-fat milk or plain low-fat yogurt

# Good news! You have only ①day to go before you binge!

## SEVENTH DAY

### BREAKFAST

¼ cup stewed apricots or prunes
½ toasted English muffin, or small blueberry or bran muffin
Thin slice swiss cheese
½ cup low-fat milk
Coffee or tea
Your vitamin SDAs

### MID-MORNING SNACK

Guilt-free snacks and beverages

### LUNCH

Salad of shredded zucchini, cabbage and sliced tomatoes
Open-faced roast beef sandwich on whole wheat bread or pumpernickel
Mint tea or club soda with lime

### MID-AFTERNOON SNACK

Guilt-free snacks and beverages

### DINNER

Mixed green salad with peppers
Oil and vinegar dressing (see first day LUNCH)
Sautéed shrimp or fillet of sole, sautéed in nonstick skillet with 1 teaspoon corn oil
½ cup each steamed or boiled cauliflower and broccoli
Fresh fruit
Mint tea or club soda with lime

### TV SNACKTIME

Guilt-free snacks and beverages

### BEDTIME SNACK

Cup low-fat milk or plain low-fat yogurt

# GUILT-FREE SNACKS AND BEVERAGES

## BEVERAGES

Coffee, preferably decaffeinated
Fruit juices, fresh, or bottled or canned
  (no sugar added), except for coconut
Soups, clear (no salt added)
Tea, regular, mint, or decaffeinated
Tomato juice (no salt added)
V-8 juice (no salt added)
Yogurt (low-fat plain)

## FRUITS

All fresh fruit, except for coconut and
  avocado

## SWEETS

Gelatin desserts (sugar-free)
Ices (sugar-free)
Sherbets (sugar-free)

## NUTS

Chestnuts

## VEGETABLES

Asparagus *
Bean sprouts
Beets *
Broccoli *
Brussels sprouts *
Cabbage **
Carrots **
Celery
Cucumbers
Cauliflower *
Endive
Green beans *
Lettuce, all types
Mushrooms
Okra *
Peppers, green and sweet red
Peas **
Popcorn (unsalted and unbuttered)
Radishes
Scallions
Spinach
Tomatoes
Turnips *
Watercress

* Items are eaten cooked, preferably steamed without salt (boiling without salt is second
  choice)

** Items are eaten cooked or raw

  Items without an * are eaten raw

  Note: For a discussion of portion sizes, see page 73.

# 10

# THE CONTROLLED BINGE WEEK: BINGE EVERY OTHER DAY AND LOSE ADDITIONAL POUNDS

You wouldn't be human if you didn't want to binge after a week on a diet, no matter how easy and pleasant the week was.

Go ahead—binge.

But binge my way.

Your appestat level will continue to lower, and you'll continue to lose weight, even though you're indulging yourself on such All-American favorites as meat and potatoes, sandwiches— and *don't* hold the mayo—veal chops, minestrone, a Western omelet, bread, muffins, margarine, cake, and even a hamburger on a bun. That's *in addition to* the satisfying food on the One-Week Crash Diet.

You won't binge just for one day in the coming week. You'll binge for *four*.

What's extraordinary about this one-week, every-other-day-binge is that you may *continue* to lose weight. You could drop from 1 to 2 pounds while you enjoy more food—and more of the food you enjoy. That could add up to *12 pounds or more lost over the first two weeks of the Vitamin Diet!*

But be aware: For some dieters, weight loss may be less than 10 pounds the first week, and less than 2 the second. Don't fret if it is. You *are* losing weight, and you *are* losing weight healthfully, and that's what matters.

## EVERY-OTHER-DAY BINGE-ING HELPS KEEP YOU ON YOUR DIET

This on-again, off-again diet relieves monotony stress—"sameness"—one of the principal reasons for going off a diet. It's easy to stay on a diet when you know that on every diet day you can look forward to a binge on the following day. What's more, on every binge day you can look forward to a completely new diet menu the next day. Variety helps keep you on your diet.

# MENUS FOR THE
# CONTROLLED
# BINGE WEEK

You can enjoy these in most restaurants, as well as in your own home. Do not cook with or add salt, sugar, butter, cream, or whole milk to any dish. Eat your salad before your entrée. Eat slowly. For super-taste sensations, use recipes from *The Vitamin Diet Gourmet Mini-Cookbook*; it starts on page 99.

# BINGE DAY

## FIRST DAY

### BREAKFAST

Half cup hot cereal of your choice, sweetened with unsweetened apple juice and cinnamon

Slice toast (preferably whole-wheat)

Teaspoon margarine (preferably made from corn oil, unsweetened, no salt added)

Cup low-fat milk

Coffee or tea

Your vitamin SDAs (see chart, page 30)

### MIDMORNING SNACK

Guilt-free snacks and beverages (see page 47)

### LUNCH

Chef salad consisting of spinach, tomatoes, cucumbers, radishes, and a small amount of cubed chicken (no bacon, please)

Up to two tablespoons salad dressing (for acceptable salad dressing for these menus, see page 199)

Small baked apple (preferably without sugar)

Coffee or tea

### MIDAFTERNOON SNACK

Guilt-free snacks and beverages

### DINNER

Alcoholic drink of your choice (optional)

Mixed green salad with tomatoes and radishes

Broiled salmon or swordfish

Cooked green beans (All cooked vegetables on these menus are preferably steamed without salt. Boiling without salt is second choice.)

Small baked potato with dollop of low-fat yogurt and minced chives or scallions

Fresh fruit cocktail

Coffee, tea, or club soda with lime

### TV SNACKTIME

Guilt-free snacks and beverages

### BEDTIME SNACK

Pleasant Dreams Snack (page 56)

---

*Note:* Binge days are not binges in the ordinary sense. They are days in which the basic healthful nutritional pattern is continued, and calories are increased moderately. Some dieters will continue to lose weight; some others will hold their weight steady. Should your scale indicate a weight gain, cut down on portion sizes on your next binge day. For calorie and sodium counts of binge day menus see page 97.

## *Good news! Tomorrow is a binge day.*

## SECOND DAY

**BREAKFAST**

Half grapefruit sweetened with spoonful of honey and sprinkled with plain toasted wheat germ
Slice French toast sprinkled with cinnamon
Coffee or tea
Your vitamin SDAs

**MIDMORNING SNACK**

Guilt-free snacks and beverages

**LUNCH**

Salad of lettuce, tomatoes, and cucumbers
Up to two tablespoons salad dressing
Open-face sandwich made with canned water-packed tuna (preferably with no salt added), sprinkled with lemon juice
Melon
Mint tea or club soda with lime

**MIDAFTERNOON SNACK**

Guilt-free snacks and beverages

**DINNER**

Tomato juice (preferably no salt added)
Salad of cucumbers, radishes, and tomatoes
Broiled chicken (without skin)
Cooked eggplant, Brussels sprouts, or turnips
Apple
Mint tea or club soda with lime

**TV SNACKTIME**

Guilt-free snacks and beverages

**BEDTIME SNACK**

Cup low-fat milk or plain low-fat yogurt

# BINGE DAY

## THIRD DAY

**BREAKFAST**

Stewed prunes
Bran muffin with
Low-fat cottage cheese (no salt added)
Coffee or tea
Your vitamin SDAs

**MIDMORNING SNACK**

Guilt-free snacks and beverages

**LUNCH**

Lettuce and tomato salad
Up to two tablespoons salad dressing
Minestrone or vegetable soup
Swiss cheese sandwich on whole-wheat
  bread
Fresh fruit salad
Coffee or tea

**MIDAFTERNOON SNACK**

Guilt-free snacks and beverages

**DINNER**

Alcoholic drink of your choice (op-
  tional)
Salad of chicory, endive, and tomatoes
Two broiled baby lamb chops or me-
  dium veal chop
Cooked carrots
Slice angel-food cake
Coffee, tea, or club soda with lime

**TV SNACKTIME**

Guilt-free snacks and beverages

**BEDTIME SNACK**

Pleasant Dreams Snack

# Good news! Tomorrow is a binge day.

## FOURTH DAY

### BREAKFAST

Orange
Shredded-wheat biscuit sprinkled with
    teaspoonful date sugar, with
Half-cup low fat milk
Coffee or tea
Your vitamin SDAs

### MIDMORNING SNACK

Guilt-free snacks and beverages

### LUNCH

Salad of shredded carrots, cabbage, and
    green peppers
Sliced turkey
Piece Melba toast
Melon
Mint tea or club soda with lime

### MIDAFTERNOON SNACK

Guilt-free snacks and beverages

### DINNER

Salad of lettuce, tomatoes, shredded raw
    zucchini, and peppers
Up to two tablespoons salad dressing
Broiled fillet of sole
Cooked asparagus, broccoli, cauliflower,
    or green beans
Fresh fruit
Mint tea or club soda with lime

### TV SNACKTIME

Guilt-free snacks and beverages

### BEDTIME SNACK

Cup low-fat milk or plain low-fat yogurt

# BINGE DAY

## FIFTH DAY

### BREAKFAST

Melon balls
Western omelet (preferably made with
  1 egg yolk, 2 egg whites, and season-
  ings; filled with sautéed peppers, on-
  ions, and tomatoes), light on the
  butter
Slice toast (preferably whole-wheat)
  with
Honey
Cup low-fat milk
Coffee or tea
Your vitamin SDAs

### MIDMORNING SNACK

Guilt-free snacks and beverages

### LUNCH

Salad of lettuce, tomatoes and boiled or
  broiled shrimp with lemon juice
One slice bread
Fresh fruit salad
Coffee or tea

### MIDAFTERNOON SNACK

Guilt-free snacks and beverages

### DINNER

Alcoholic drink of your choice (op-
  tional)
Mixed green salad
Salad dressing
Broiled sirloin steak with onions
Slice angel-food cake
Coffee, tea, or club soda with lime

### TV SNACKTIME

Guilt-free snacks and beverages

### BEDTIME SNACK

Pleasant Dreams Snack

## Good news! Tomorrow is a binge day.

## SIXTH DAY

### BREAKFAST

Orange
Half cup hot oatmeal or Wheatena sweetened with unsweetened apple juice, sprinkled with plain toasted wheat germ
Half-cup low-fat milk
Coffee or tea
Your vitamin SDAs

### MIDMORNING SNACK

Guilt-free snacks and beverages

### LUNCH

Consommé
Salad of cucumbers, green peppers, and radishes
Open-face Jarlsberg cheese sandwich (whole-wheat bread preferred)
Mint tea or club soda with lime

### MIDAFTERNOON SNACK

Guilt-free snacks and beverages

### DINNER

Tomato juice (preferably no salt added)
Mixed green salad with green peppers
Up to two tablespoons salad dressing
Roast chicken (without skin)
Cooked asparagus, broccoli, or cauliflower
Canned pineapple in its own juice
Mint tea or club soda with lime

### TV SNACKTIME

Guilt-free snacks and beverages

### BEDTIME SNACK

Cup low-fat milk or plain low-fat yogurt

# BINGE DAY!

## SEVENTH DAY

### BREAKFAST

Fresh fruit cup
Scrambled egg cooked in nonstick skillet
    with 1 teaspoon corn oil or margarine
    (preferably from corn oil, unsweet-
    ened, no salt added)
Bran or whole-wheat muffin
Coffee or tea
Your vitamin SDAs

### MIDMORNING SNACK

Guilt-free snacks and beverages

### LUNCH

Salad of lettuce and tomatoes
Broiled hamburger on bun
Melon
Coffee or tea

### MIDAFTERNOON SNACK

Guilt-free snacks and beverages

### DINNER

Alcoholic drink of your choice (op-
    tional)
Salad of endive and arrugula
Up to two tablespoons salad dressing
Broiled mixed seafood plate (your
    choice)
Small baked potato with dollop of low-
    fat yogurt and minced chives or scal-
    lions
Small baked apple (preferably without
    sugar)
Coffee, tea, or club soda with lime

### TV SNACKTIME

Guilt-free snacks and beverages

### BEDTIME SNACK

Pleasant Dreams Snack

# A SPECIAL TREAT TO PAMPER YOUR SWEET TOOTH

### PLEASANT DREAMS SNACK

Place 1 tablespoon puffed wheat (no sugar added) or 4 spoon-size shredded wheat biscuits in dessert cup. Add 1 tea-spoon honey. Pour in ½ cup ice-cold low-fat milk. What a sweet way to end a day!

# 11

# HOW TO STICK TO YOUR DIET WHEN YOU EAT OUT

Eating in restaurants, which spells disaster on most other diets, is a simple, pleasant experience on mine.

That's *so* important to you. If you're like most working dieters, you eat five to 10 meals a week away from home. You want to be sure when you go on a diet that your regular eating-out patterns won't be disturbed. They *won't* on this diet.

This revolutionary Vitamin Diet is a practical diet, designed with your eating-out needs in mind. There's nothing on it that you can't get in most restaurants. You'll never again have to brown-paper-bag it; never again have to say, "I'm sorry, I can't eat out with you, I'm on a diet"; never again have to feel like an outsider at a business lunch. All you have to do in a restaurant is order your meals exactly as they appear on my diet menus.

To get the most out of restaurant dining, follow these simple—

## DO'S AND DON'TS FOR DIETING OUT ENJOYABLY

*Do* carry with you each day's Vitamin Diet Menu. You can clip them from this book, copy them, or Xerox them. *Don't* trust to your memory.

*Do* order your three major meals from your day's safe and sure Diet Menu. *Don't* order from the restaurant menu. Don't even look at it. Why let yourself be tempted by all those fabulously fattening dishes?

*Do* use common sense when the waiter says, "Sorry, but we're all out of . . ." something or other on the day's Diet Menu. If, for example, you can't get an endive or arugula salad (you can in many Italian restaurants), order a mixed green salad instead.

*Do* select your bread quota, then ask your waiter to remove the bread basket. A filled bread basket is the single most dangerous anti-diet weapon ever invented. *Don't* fall back on that dieter's alibi, "Oh, I'm paying for it, I might as well eat it."

*Do* ask the waiter to remove your salt shaker, condiments, and pickles. Remember, salt can put on more weight (in water) than a low-calorie meal can take off (in fat). *Don't* just use "a little salt," or "some" condiments, or "just a slice of" pickle. Salted food stimulates the appetite; and once you start, you'll find it hard to stop. That's why the first person who eats only *one* commercial potato chip deserves a place in the *Guinness Book of Records.*

*Do* ask how the vegetables are prepared. If they're steamed, boiled, or sautéed with vegetable oil, and no salt is added, fine. If they're made to order, instruct the waiter, "No salt, please. Ask the chef to use herbs and spices instead." It works for me every time. *Don't* order fried vegetables, breaded vegetables, or vegetables served with sauce. Avoid gooey vegetable casseroles as well. And, if the waiter answers "Yes" to "Are they cooked with butter?" respond with a "No."

*Do* eat your potatoes baked or boiled. Baked is preferred because the skin is richer in nutrients than the body, and no chef adds salt to a baked potato. Chances are you can't get a boiled potato that isn't at least lightly salted, unless it's made to order. If it is, request, "No salt, please." *Don't* be tempted by French fries, home fries, mashed potatoes, *pommes soufflé*, potatoes Anna, Lyonnaise potatoes, potatoes au gratin, and other gussied-up potatoes that blow you up.

*Do* order your baked potato plain (if it's an Idaho, it's sheer heaven that way), or sparked with a dollop of low-fat yogurt and chives or scallions, or sprinkled with ground red (cayenne) pepper. *Don't*, when the waiter asks, "Sour cream or butter?" choose either. (I've heard some overweights answer, "Both.")

*Do* order only salads made from plain greens, fruits, or vegetables. Raw, of course; but blanched vegetables may be used on occasions. Eat as is, or bring out the flavor of the food with lemon juice, or oil and vinegar dressing. Be wary of prepared oil and vinegar dressings;

they're probably loaded with salt. Play it safe and ask for separate containers of oil and vinegar, and mix your own dressing—but easy on the oil. *Don't* order potato salad, cole slaw, cucumber salad, Greek salad, chef's salad, or mushroom and bacon salad. They're heavy in fat and salt, and some contain large quantities of sugar as well. For the same reason, and because all contain large quantities of sugar, avoid French dressing, Russian dressing, cheese dressings, Italian dressing, and other restaurant standbys including house dressings.

*Do* order your salad, and eat it, before your main course. (Most restaurants serve it in that order anyway.) A salad fills you up without filling you out, and you eat less of the higher-caloric entrée. *Don't* consider your salad as a side dish. It's less slimming eaten that way.

*Do* order your entrée without sauce, even when the waiter insists that the chef always makes it *with* sauce. The chef is there to please you; and even if the dish is pre-prepared, he can easily remove the sauce. It's wise to avoid the sauce because it contains all that fat, salt, and sugar. *Don't* order the sauce on the side "just for a taste." Sauces (except mine) are appetite stimulants. Just what you *don't* want on a diet.

*Do* order, preferably, simple roasted, baked, grilled, or broiled meats, fish, and poultry. Tell the waiter—and here it comes again—"No salt, please. But see what the chef can do with herbs and spices." *Don't* accept the waiter's, "Leave it to me. I'll bring you something you'll like." The chances are you won't like it. Warn him, "Listen, if there's sauce on it, or if it's salty, I'm going to send it back."

*Do*, if your food is being made to order, ask the waiter to have the chef trim away all visible fat before cooking, and to cook without grease or salt. *Don't* skip making this request because you think you're making waves. Ask for what you want and you'll get it. Practical hint: Grease the waiter's palm with a bit more than the customary 15 percent tip, and you'll have no trouble getting grease-free, and salt-free, cooking the next time around.

*Do* perk up your fish and seafood dishes with juice freshly squeezed from lemon wedges. It enhances the natural flavors. *Don't* let the waiter browbeat you into accepting sauces or melted butter. They mask flavors as well as put weight on you.

*Do* take your vitamin SDAs after your meal (preferably after breakfast). *Don't* be embarrassed by taking "pills" in public. More and more vitamin-conscious Americans are doing just that. It's for the sake of your health and good looks. Flaunt it!

*Do*, if you're a steady customer, refer the manager to the mouth-watering *The Vitamin Diet Gourmet Mini-Cookbook* which begins on page 99, or to any of my other nationally acclaimed cookbooks. Ask him to follow my recipes for you. *Don't* think you're offending him. A rising trend toward cooking for better health is sweeping the nation, and he'll want to get on the bandwagon. You won't be the only customer for whom he'll be preparing delicious slimming food. He'll thank you.

# 12

# SELECTING THE BEST KINDS OF RESTAURANTS IN WHICH TO DIET

My husband and I, food connoisseurs all our adult lives, have over the last eight years ranked the kinds of restaurants available to most Americans in terms of how well you can diet in them. Here are the results.

One star (★) means they're good places in which to diet; two stars (★★) mean they're very good; and three stars (★★★) mean they're excellent. No star means you're taking a risk.

*Airliners.* During some flights, airliners become restaurants, serving, in addition to their regular fare, kosher, vegetarian, low-sodium, low-fat, low-cholesterol, low-calorie, and diabetic meals (provided you place your order 24 hours in advance). You can't stay on *this* diet on an airliner, but you can continue to diet on the low-calorie meals. But if you've ever eaten 60,000 feet into the wild blue yonder, you know the food, tastewise, never gets off the ground.

★★★ *American restaurants.* No problems in expensive ones (they'll steam your vegetables, and replace salt with herbs and spices), minor problems in moderate-priced ones (vegetables are usually sautéed or boiled instead of steamed, and chefs lack skill with herbs and spices).

*Cafeterias.* Not for us. Sugar, grease, and salt abound. You *can* get fresh fruit.But unless you're on a kookie diet, who would want to live on fruit alone?

*Chinese restaurants.* Some of the dishes on my diet menus can be done Chinese style (there are many such recipes in my other books), but it is doubtful whether a Chinese restaurant chef would bother. You *can* get lovely steamed vegetables, fish, and other delectables, but in most Chinese restaurants you'll have a hassle about leaving off salt, soy sauce, and MSG. MSG and soy sauce are high in sodium, the water-retaining, appetite-stimulating element in salt.

*Coffee shops.* Don't go, except to some for breakfast. It saddens me that so many coffee shops do not serve low-fat, nonfat, or skim milk.

*Chain restaurants.* See Institutional restaurants.

★★★ *East European restaurants.* Provided your food is made to your specifications, you're in for a treat. The chefs of Hungary, Czechoslovakia, and the Balkans are adept in the use of herbs and spices, so vital when cooking without salt. But stay clear of their regular dishes.

*Fast food joints.*  Skip.

*French restaurants (classic style).* The chefs can cook my haute cuisine of health style on request, but did you ever have a captain look down his nose at you? Not worth the indignity, not to mention the $40-or-so per person price tab. Classic French food—replete with egg yolks, cream, animal fats, sugar, and salt—is the richest in the world.

★ *French restaurants (cuisine minceur or nouvelle cuisine style).* They cut down on fattening no-nos, but don't replace them with tasteful yes-yesses (as I do). If you can put up with a bland meal, your diet won't suffer here.

*Health food restaurants.* Predominantly vegetarian, they offer little to my kind of dieter. Their regular food is heavily salted, buttered, sugared, and fatted. You can get a *plain* broiled fish, and a *plain* salad, if you fight for it. But why eat out on tasteless food, particularly when you're on a diet?

★★★ *Hotel (de luxe) restaurants.* You can get anything you want prepared the way you want it. The chefs will make valiant attempts to please your palate when you order from my diet menus. Excellent for breakfasts.

★★ *Hotel (moderate-priced) restaurants.* My diet food is not prepared as well as in deluxe hotel restaurants, but the fare ranges from good to excellent. Breakfasts can be every bit as good as in deluxe restaurants, but you may have a job getting salt-free cereals.

*Institutional restaurants.* These include school and hospital restaurants, employee cafeterias, chain restaurants, motel restaurants, and even executive-suite restaurants. They are supplied by the institutional food industry with mass-produced convenience foods, which are simply heated, then served. They include massive amounts of salt, sugar, and fat. No, or very little, chance here of diet foods made to your order.

★★★ *Italian restaurants.* When the chef cooperates and adds the right amount of herbs and spices of his native land to compensate for saltlessness, you'll want to cry "bellissimo!" Our favorites.

*Japanese restaurants.* As in Chinese restaurants, the food is low in calories, but beware the salt. (In Japan salt consumption is higher than in any other nation, and so is the rate of high blood pressure.) A Japanese chef could convert some of the dishes on my diet menus to his way of cooking, but they would be tasteless without soy sauce (which is a virtually saturated solution of salt). Besides, I don't think he'd want to. Japanese restaurants are not for you. So sorry.

*Motel restaurants.* See Institutional restaurants.

★★★ *Seafood and fish restaurants.* No trouble at all getting the food prepared exactly the way you order it. Some restaurants of this type work wonders with herbs and spices. Highly recommended.

★ *Steak houses.* For your meat meals. They rate only one star because the best of them use only prime meats, which are the fattiest, and the chefs have only minimal skills in the use of herbs and spices. The cheaper steak houses use choice meats, which are diet acceptable, but you'll have a hard time rounding out a complete diet meal in them.

# 13

# THE THIN-FOR-LIFE PROGRAM

Dr. Robert C. Atkins tells his patients, so he reports, that "Any idiot can *lose* weight—it's staying thin that's the test!"

Wrong. And right.

*Wrong* because losing weight is not the work of "any idiot." It's an accomplishment of a person wise enough to know that shedding weight means becoming more attractive, more employable, and healthier.

*Right* because keeping off lost weight is virtually impossible for most people. If you've dieted before you wouldn't be reading this book if you hadn't put it back on. How long did it take you to look the way you did before you took it off—a year? a few months? a week? a *day?*

You're not alone. Dr. Norman Jolliffe, that medical genius upon whose work my pathbreaking Vitamin Diet is based, wrote, "Ninety percent of people who successfully reduce, regain sooner or later—more sooner than later—their weight." That figure has been updated to at least 95 percent. Drs. A. J. Stunkard and M. McLaren Home studied medical weight-loss statistics over a 30-year span and concluded, "Most [permanent] attempts to control overweight have been ineffective."

Why?

"Because," answered Dr. Jolliffe, "[dieters] have not learned appetite control and elementary dietetics."

But *you* have.

And you've learned it the best way—by doing.

*You've learned* how to help regulate your appetite-control mechanism, your appestat, by supplementing one meal a day with your Slimming Daily Allowances (your SDAs) of vitamins and RDAs of minerals.

*You've learned* how to avoid appetite-stimulant nutrients—sugar, salt, and excess fat—which raise the level of the appestat and cause you to overeat.

*You've learned* how to add high-fiber foods to your diet to avoid between-meals hunger pangs, which also reset the appestat too high.

*You've learned*, from following my menus, to live on a *balanced* diet—the right amounts of carbohydrates, proteins, fats, minerals, and vitamins—to keep your appestat functioning at its normal level.

Now what you've learned will go to work *for* you as you follow these—

# SEVEN SIMPLE RULES FOR STAYING THIN FOR LIFE

1. As you grow older, adjust your SDAs for your age group (see chart, page 30).
2. Do not add salt and sugar to your food either at the table or in the kitchen, and avoid canned, frozen, and prepared food with high hidden salt and sugar content.
3. Be sure your foods are low in fat, and remove all visible fat from them, preferably before cooking. Remove other fat during cooking, and at the table.
4. Balance your diet by following the healthful and tasteful Thin-for-Life Menu Plan, which begins on page 66. You can enjoy the meals in most restaurants, as well as in your own home.
5. Select specific ingredients for the Thin-for-Life Menu Plan from the list of Yes-Yes Foods beginning on page 101.
6. Brighten your meals at home with recipes from *The Vitamin Diet Gourmet Mini-Cookbook* (pages 99–198).

   And, most important—
7. Eat as much as you like, and, in the words of Dr. Jolliffe, "trust your appestat" to prevent yourself from overeating.

# HOW TO GET THE MOST FROM YOUR THIN-FOR-LIFE MENU PLAN

For peak health and permanent slimness, follow these simple guidelines:
• Do not eat meat more than twice a week.
• Do not eat meat on successive days.
• Do not eat meat more than once a day.
• Alternate meat days, fish days, and poultry days.
• Set aside one day a week for vegetarian meals.
• Do not eat more than three eggs a week.
• Do not eat more than one egg in a day.
• Do not eat eggs on successive days.
• Eat your salad before your entrée.
• In place of commercial condiments, use appropriately at table or in the kitchen herbs and spices, garlic, onion, shallots, lemon and lime juices, and my salad dressings (see pages 161–63).
• Do not eat pickles or pickled or smoked foods.

  And—
• Expand the joys of the table with my haute cuisine of health recipes—no sugar, no salt, low fat, low saturated fat, low cholesterol, high fiber.

# THE THIN-FOR-LIFE MENU PLAN

*Eat as much as you like and trust your appestat.*

# BREAKFAST

## FRUIT

Any in season except coconut or avocado. Eat raw or cooked, using unsweetened apple juice, a small amount of honey, or date sugar as a sweetener.

*or*

## FRUIT JUICE

Any except coconut.

## CEREALS

Any whole grain or enriched, hot or cold, no sugar or salt added. Use nonfat milk. Add fresh fruit if desired and/or sprinkle with wheat germ and unprocessed bran.

## EGGS

Any style, boiled or poached preferred. Make French toast using only half egg yolk and 2 egg whites to serve two.

*or*

## TOFU

*(bean curd)*, any style, without soy sauce.

*or*

## COTTAGE CHEESE

less than ½ percent milk fat, no salt added. Use as main dish with fruit, or lightly sweetened with honey and sprinkled with wheat germ.

*or*

## PLAIN LOW-FAT YOGURT

as is, or with fresh fruit, or sweetened with a small amount of honey.

## BREAD

Whole-wheat, or enriched French and Italian, or my bread (it's the most delicious and nutritious; recipes on pages 150–55). Serve as is or toasted.

## MARGARINE

Sweet (unsalted) 100 percent corn oil, spread thin (it tastes better that way).

*or*

## COTTAGE CHEESE

less than ½ percent milk fat, no salt added. Use as a spread.

## JELLIES AND JAMS

Any honey-sweetened.

## BEVERAGES

Coffee or tea, decaffeinated preferred; or coffee substitutes such as Cafix (look for it and others like it in health food stores); or any mint tea. Sweeten if desired with small amounts of honey, or enhance flavor with lemon peel and/or cinnamon stick. Low-fat, no-fat, or skim milk may be added. You can also enjoy these kinds of milk as your beverage. Plain low-fat yogurt is also acceptable.

## VITAMINS

Your SDAs.

# *Eat as much as you like and trust your appestat.*

## LUNCH

### FRUIT

*See* Breakfast.

*or*

### FRUIT JUICE

*See* Breakfast.

*or*

### VEGETABLE JUICE

Any, such as tomato juice or V-8, no salt added.

### SALADS

Any mixed green.

*or*

### CRUDITÉS

(colorfully arranged raw vegetables).

*or*

### BLANCHED COLD VEGETABLES

Such as broccoli, zucchini, Brussels sprouts, or carrots, or any combination.

### SALAD DRESSINGS

Oil and vinegar, lemon, or my zesty salad dressings (see pages 161–63).

### SOUPS

Any, except those made with cream, whole milk, or whole yogurt (salt-free preferred).

### SANDWICHES

Fillings from any entrée, or from the following delicatessen foods: roast beef, chicken, and turkey. For breads, *see* Breakfast.

### ENTRÉES

Any lean meat, fish, or fowl (white meat preferred), hot or cold. Alternates: Fruit salad with cottage cheese (less than ½ percent milk fat, no salt added); tofu prepared any way, without soy sauce; low-fat plain yogurt with fresh fruit, sweetened with a small amount of honey, if desired. A sandwich and soup or a sandwich and salad may take the place of an entrée and a starchy vegetable.

### VEGETABLES

One dark green vegetable, preferably steamed; and one starchy vegetable such as corn, rice, lima beans, or potato (baked or boiled). Fresh vegetables are preferred to frozen. Canned vegetables (except dietetic pack) are prohibited because of their high salt content.

## BREAD

Two slices *(see* Breakfast), unless used in a sandwich.

## DESSERTS

Fresh fruit or canned pineapple packed in its own juice. Sherbets, ices, and gelatin desserts, sugar-free, can also be enjoyed.

## BEVERAGES

*See* Breakfast. Any low-sodium mineral water, such as Perrier, can be enjoyed instead of, or in addition to, the other beverages. A slice of lime adds flavor.

## *Eat as much as you like and trust your appestat.*

# DINNER

**PRE-DINNER DRINK (OPTIONAL)**

Just one. Or a glass of wine with your
  meal.

**SEA FOOD COCKTAIL**

*or*

**CRUDITÉS**

*See* Lunch.

*or*

**FRESH FRUIT COCKTAIL**

*or*

**BITE-SIZE CHEESE CUBES**

(low-fat cheese preferred).

*or*

**MY HORS D'OEUVRES**

(See pages 169–73.)

**SALADS**

*See* Lunch.

**SOUPS**

*See* Lunch.

**ENTRÉES**

Any lean meat, fish, or fowl (light meat
  preferred), hot or cold. Alternates:
  Pasta, no salt added, preferably with
  unsalted sauce; fish salads; any vegetable dish.

**VEGETABLES**

*See* Lunch. But omit starchy vegetable
  if you're having pasta.

**BREAD**

*See* Lunch. But omit if you're having
  pasta.

**MARGARINE**

*See* Lunch.

**DESSERTS**

Mine (See pages 189–94), plus angel-
  food cake; *see also* Lunch.

**BEVERAGES**

*See* Lunch.

*Eat as much as you like and trust your appestat.*

## SNACKS

To be consumed slowly midmorning, midafternoon, TV snacktime, and bedtime.

Add to Guilt-Free Snacks (see page 47) and Pleasant Dreams Snack (page 56), raisins and walnuts (or almonds); dates, figs, or prunes, or any combination; dried pineapples, papaya, apricots, pears, or peaches (no sugar added), or any combination; rice wafers or wheat wafers (salt-free); all fruit juices (sugar-free) except coconut.

---

*Note:* It takes at least four to six weeks to normalize your appestat. If you've reached ideal weight before four to six weeks, follow this procedure:

Multiply your weight by 10, then by 15. That gives you a rough calorie range per day for keeping your weight steady.

Then prepare the menus in this chapter to provide those calories and no more. Get the calorie counts from the chart beginning on page 101. After four weeks of reducing and maintenance dieting, begin to experiment with trusting your appestat.

# PART III

## MAKING THIS DIET WORK *FOR* YOU —MORE RAPIDLY AND HEALTHFULLY

# 14

# EVERYTHING YOU ALWAYS WANTED TO KNOW ABOUT REDUCING AND STAYING REDUCED BUT NEVER KNEW WHO TO ASK

I have made recently more than 300 appearances on radio and TV and before lecture groups in cities, towns, and suburbs across the nation discussing the health, nutritional, and gastronomic aspects of my diet. The questions that appear throughout this book are those most frequently asked by people like yourself. In this chapter, you'll find answers to questions about the overall diet; in the next chapter, answers to questions about vitamins.

## CLEARING UP DETAILS THAT COULD TRIP YOU UP

*What do I do if I can't find a prescribed food, or I'm allergic to it, or I don't want to spend the money for it, or I just don't like it?*

Use your common sense and substitute an equivalent food. The list of Yes-Yes Foods (page 101) can be of help to you. But remember, sticking rigorously to an inflexible diet is a behavior-conditioning mechanism to help you acquire long-lasting slimming and healthful eating habits.

*You give portion sizes for some dishes and not for others. Why?*

It's a good idea to start trusting your appestat with the dishes to which I don't assign portion sizes. There's no danger of hurting your weight-reducing effort unless you deliberately set out to stuff yourself. The reason is that on the reducing diet your appestat level is lower than it was before you started dieting, so when you eat until your appestat sends out its enough-is-enough signal, you'll be eating less than before and will still lose weight. Also, the dishes with unassigned portion sizes are mostly entrées, and about one kind of entrée, Dr. Jolliffe wrote, "A curious nutritional fact is on your side. No one is able to eat enough *lean* meat *alone* to gain weight; it is the French fries, the beer, and the pie that go with it that do the damage." It is reasonable to assume that other high-protein entrées—fish, chicken, and turkey—are similarly safe.

However, if you feel uneasy at this stage about trusting your appestat, follow these rules: For entrées: 2 ounces for lunch and 3 ounces for dinner for most women and small-frame men; and 2 ounces for lunch and 4 ounces for dinner for most men and large-frame women. For vegetables: half-cups. For non-caloric beverages: no limit (but it would be wise to keep your coffee and tea down to 2 cups a day). For caloric beverages: one 6-ounce serving. For guilt-free snacks: one small serving. For sweets: one small serving. Four chestnuts. And all the salad you can eat, but do *not* increase the assigned amount of dressing.

A good supplementary guide to portion sizes on a Jolliffe-type diet is *Eat to Lose Weight*. It's free from the Bureau of Nutrition, New York City Department of Health, 93 Worth Street, Room 714, New York, N.Y. 10013.

*I notice you prefer toast and whole-wheat bread. Is that because they have less calories than untoasted and regular bread?*

No, the calorie counts are about the same. I prefer whole-wheat bread because it's high in fiber. (It's no richer in vitamin content than some enriched white breads.) Toast gets my nod of approval because of its warmth and taste. If your taste runs to untoasted bread, by all means have it.

*Prepared diet food is now available in so many varieties, but I don't see any of it on your menus. Why?*

I've made this point often: Most people can't stay on a diet unless the food is familiar and tastes good. Much prepared diet food is seasoned with salt substitutes and sweetened with sugar substitutes, both of which are alien to the palate and taste *ugh*-ly. Some prepared diet foods are manufactured without any added flavorings, and are so different from your regular fare, and so blah, that you feel you're being punished every time you take a forkful. Diet food should be delicious, not dull; exciting, not depressing.

Must *I* eat everything?
*Everything!* Each item on a menu contributes its share of the nutrients your

body needs to function efficiently. Skip one item, and your diet is nutrient-deficient. That's a health hazard. It's also a weight-loss hazard. When there's a nutrient deficiency in your meal, your appestat resets at a higher level in an attempt to make up the deficiency with more food. Eat just one dish less, and you'll eat more of the remaining dishes than you should.

*Avocados and coconuts are popular among many people concerned with their health. Why do you put them on your no-no list?*

They're high in fat, and very high in saturated fat (the kind of fat that can clog your arteries and hurt you in other ways).

*If it's okay to eat honey and date sugar, why can't I eat regular sugar?*

Regular sugar (sucrose) has been associated with degenerative diseases by some medical authorities; honey and date sugar have not. Regular sugar is an empty-calorie food—it contains no vitamins or minerals, just calories. Honey is a solution of mainly glucose and fructose, and has many verified health-promoting qualities. Date sugar is not sugar at all, but pulverized crushed dates. It is sometimes known as "date powder."

*Eggs are said to be the perfect food, yet you use them sparingly. Why?*

An egg yolk contains about 250 milligrams of cholesterol, a fat-related substance that could be a cause of atherosclerosis (thickening of the arteries) and subsequent heart attack. A safe daily intake of cholesterol ranges from 160 to 185 milligrams. For the sake of your health, it's wise to limit egg yolks to three a week. Egg whites, though, are A-OK.

*A calorie, I understand, is really a measure of heat. So if I eat cold foods, am I taking in less calories than if I eat hot foods?*

If the answer were yes, you can be sure somebody would have invented the Cold Food Diet—Reduce Fast on Ice Cream, Vichyssoise, and Ice Cubes. A calorie, in the physiological sense, is a measure of the heat generated by burning food in the body to supply energy (much as coal is burned in a furnace). Whether the food is hot or cold, the same amount of calories is produced. Eating cold food is of no advantage to the dieter.

# GUIDELINES FOR LOSING WEIGHT EVEN FASTER

*I'm told that 25 percent of the fat in a chicken is in the skin. Is that true?*

It is. And that's why it's diet-wise to remove the skin before cooking; or, if you're dining out, remove it before eating.

*I know enough to cut away all visible fat from my meat. But what do I do about the fat that I can't see?*

Broil, roast, grill, or rotiss. The fat drips off. Same advice goes for poultry and fat fish.

*I notice an absence of condiments on your diet. But mustard, catsup, steak sauce, and soy sauce have only 15 calories per tablespoon. And on other diets I've been told I could eat all the pickles I wanted because they're so low in calories. Are these oversight on your part?*

No way. Pickles and condiments *are* low in calories, but they're screamingly high in salt. Salt holds on to water, and water is heavy—you know the old jingle, "A pint's a pound the world around." The salt in just one dill pickle holds on to more than two pounds of water! Banish condiments when you're dieting and your excess water will flow off faster.

*Did you exclude liquor on your One-Week Crash Diet because it stimulates the appetite?*

No. The appetite-stimulating properties of alcohol have been grossly exaggerated. (In excess, though, it does release inhibitions, and you could reach for more food than you should.) I eliminated alcohol because it's an empty-calorie food (a food with no nutrient value). And on a crash diet, which is low in calories, you need all the nutrient value you can get to feel not just as good as before, but better. You can enjoy dry (not sweet) alcoholic drinks on the other parts of my total diet program.

*A friend told me if I eat slowly I'll lose weight faster. That seems strange to me.*

Not so strange if you look at it this way. It takes time before your meal digests and affects your appestat. Let's say it takes 30 minutes. At that time the enough's-enough signal goes off, and you feel filled up. But suppose you finish your meal in 15 minutes. There's no signal from the appestat, and you go right on eating. By the time 30 minutes are up, you've eaten two meals instead of one. Is it a wonder so many overweights are fast eaters? *Slow down and slim down.*

*I hear that if I chew my food thoroughly I'll lose weight faster. Can you tell me—is that true?*

It is. Eating slowly helps prevent you from overeating, and the best way to eat slowly is to chew thoroughly. Chew until every bit of flavor has been removed from each mouthful—and that takes time.

*I've never used chopsticks. I've heard I can lose weight faster if I learn how to use them, and practice on my diet meals. What do you think?*

It's gimmicky, even though the idea behind it is sound: it slows up your eating time, and *that* does help you lose weight faster. But there are other "tricks"— actually behavioral training patterns developed by medical and psychological weight-reduction specialists—that can help you reduce faster without learning new skills. They work by replacing your old overeating habits with new normal-eating ones. They can help you reduce rapidly and stay reduced permanently. Here are the best of them:

# HOW—NOT WHAT—TO EAT TO LOSE WEIGHT FASTER AND KEEP IT OFF

• *Eat only at specific times.* Set specific times for your three major meals and four snacks. TV snacktime should be set, for example, from 9:10 to 9:20, or from 9:30 to 9:40, and not continue from prime time to the late, late show. Eat at your set times, and in a short time you'll have no desire to eat between times.

• *Eat only at a specific place in your home.* Preferably, that should be a place at your dining table. Reason: Otherwise you'd eat in your bedroom, your reading chair, your workroom, and so on. That's an open invitation to unending snacking. One exception to the specific-place rule: You may also eat in front of the tube during your specific TV snacktime.

• *Eat restaurant-style at home.* You'll find one serving is enough. Family-style servings tempt you to seconds, thirds, fourths. . . .

• *Eat all your meals.* Skip one meal, and you'll overeat on the next one. Eating three major meals and four snacks a day also has this advantage: it keeps you energetic all day long. An airplane needs a constant supply of fuel to keep flying. So do you.

• *Eat only what's in front of you.* Don't go rushing off to the fridge or your cupboards for more. When you snack, fill the bowl with assigned portions or just enough goodies to satisfy your appestat. You'll get to know by experience just how much that is.

• *Shop on a full stomach, and carry a shopping list.* That's the way to avoid overstocking, and stocking up on no-nos.

• *Eat without distractions.* Ever get up from a night before the tube and exclaim, "Did I eat *all that!*"? If you don't keep your mind on what you eat, you'll never mind how much you eat.

And, most important—

• *Eat slowly.* Here are some hints to help you master the art of slow eating. It's an art practiced by gourmets to savor the full flavors of foods.

—Place only one kind of food in your mouth at a time. Eat a bit of potato, *then* a bit of steak. That takes two times as long as eating the bits of steak and potato together.

—Cut your food into bite-size or less-than-bite-size pieces. Cutting takes time; and it takes more time to eat many small pieces than it does to eat one large piece.

—Set down your eating utensils after you've placed your food in your mouth. It takes time to set them down, and it takes time to pick them up.

—Take a time out between courses. That not only slows you down, but, food lovers will tell you, makes the next course taste better.

—Fill your mealtimes with pleasant conversation. When you talk, you don't eat. That makes the meal last longer.

—And, most important, chew, chew, chew!

*I'm a cookie junkie. If there's a box of cookies in the house when I get home from work, I'll eat every last one of them before I go to bed. What's the remedy?*
The night before you start on this diet, get rid of every cookie in the house. Give them away, throw them away—get rid of them any way except devouring them. Don't leave a cookie crumb behind. And don't buy another cookie for the duration of the diet. The same rule applies to all other fattening foods.

*I don't ordinarily exercise. But I will if it will help me lose weight faster. Will it?*
It *will*. I'll tell you everything a dieter should know about exercise in Chapter 16.

## HOW THIS DIET SIDESTEPS THE HARMFUL SIDE EFFECTS OF FAD DIETS

*When I dieted before, people told me I had bad breath. Was that my fault or the diet's?*
The diet's. Very high-protein and high-fat diets can produce ketosis, a pathological condition associated with diabetes. One of the symptoms of that disease is bad breath—the sickly sweet odor of acetone. This is a moderate-protein and low-fat diet. It cannot produce ketosis.

*On one diet I went on, I got constipation, on another diet diarrhea. Will I get either on your diet?*
Your elimination problems were caused by unbalanced diets—an excess of some nutrients, a deficiency of others. One fad-diet doctor actually prescribed laxatives with his diet! This diet is balanced, and causes neither constipation nor diarrhea.

*One crash diet I was on required me to drink eight glasses of water a day. How many glasses of water are required on your diet?*
On that diet, you *had* to drink that amount of water to wash out of your body poisons generated by the diet—probably uric acid and/or ketones. No poisons are generated by this diet, so you only have to drink enough water to satisfy your thirst.

*I'm always so crabby when I diet. Must I expect more of the same on your diet?*
No. As a matter of fact, you'll feel full of life. Your crabbiness came from hunger pangs and probably from vitamin B starvation. There are no hunger pangs on this diet because you eat enough to satisfy your appestat, and your diet is supplemented with an adequate amount of vitamin B.

# 15

# ANSWERS TO YOUR QUESTIONS ABOUT VITAMINS AND DIET

*Your diet is an update and upgrade of Dr. Norman Jolliffe's medically acclaimed diet. Did Dr. Jolliffe prescribe vitamin supplements?*
Of course. But back in 1958–62, when his diet was tested, the nation's diet was not as vitamin impoverished as it is now. He needed to supplement his diet with only moderate quantities of eight vitamins. It is now necessary to add optimal quantities of 15 of the known 18 vitamins. Jolliffe had no "vitamin diet."

*What's the difference between RDAs and SDAs?*
RDAs are the Recommended Daily Allowances of vitamins estimated by the Food and Nutrition Board of the National Research Council. The Food and Drug Administration uses these estimates as a basis for its standards for vitamin consumption, called U.S. RDAs. Food labels often list percentages of U.S. RDAs per serving or container. When your daily vitamin intake matches U.S. RDAs, you can be reasonably sure of protection against vitamin-deficiency diseases such as scurvy, rickets, pellagra, and beri-beri.

SDAs (Slimming Daily Allowances) are a composite of recommendations based on the work of many vitamin experts. They represent the amounts of vitamins that not only afford protection against vitamin-deficiency diseases but also keep your body operating at peak efficiency. They are in most cases somewhat higher than RDAs, and in the case of vitamin C and the B complex vitamins, considerably higher.

*I was taught in school that a balanced diet such as yours contains all the vitamins I need. I don't understand why I need supplements.*
There was a time when a balanced diet *did* supply sufficient quantities of all 18 vitamins. But that was before food processing and the contemporary lifestyle. Today, observes Dr. Mark O. Hegsted of the U.S. Department of Agriculture, it is not at all likely that you can meet several RDA vitamin requirements with your knife and fork unless you consume more than 2,000 calories a day.

*Is lack of sufficient quantities of vitamins in our diet the reason that about half of the adults in this country are overweight?*
It's one reason. The appestat is set high to bring in a greater amount of food than is necessary in an attempt (which often fails) to supply the body with suffi-

cient quantities of vitamins to operate at peak efficiency. Another reason for our epidemic of obesity is the great amounts of appetite stimulants with little or no nutritional value—salt, sugar, and excess fat—processed into our foods. At least half of the nation is undernourished and overfed.

### Do your SDAs for vitamin products give me all the vitamins I need to help me stay slim and healthy?

The SDAs for vitamin products represent general guidelines. Every one of us is different, and every one of us needs a different amount of vitamins. The chart on the following page, based on the work of Dr. Michael Feldzamen and other vitamin investigators, indicates optimal quantity range for each of the supplementary 15 vitamins you require for peak health. You can vary the quantities within each range until you find the amounts that are best for you as evidenced by your overall feeling of well-being. But before experimenting, consult your physician.

### Do I need to use Your Individual Vitamin SDAs chart when I go on this diet?

No. The three kinds of vitamin products I suggest in the chart Your Slimming Daily Allowances of Vitamins (page 30) contain sufficient quantities of all 15 vitamins to satisfy the needs of most people. (The potencies of the vitamins in the products on that chart roughly meet the standards of the Your Individual Vitamin SDAs chart.)

### Must I take all three kinds of vitamin products?

Yes. Although every vitamin has a specific function, all work together as a team. Deleting a vitamin or decreasing its potency adversely affects the performances of all vitamins.

### Must I take vitamin supplements every day on your Thin-for-Life maintenance diet?

Yes. Many vitamin experts agree that vitamin supplementation must be comprehensive, consistent, and continuous.

### Must I take my vitamins with a meal?

Your body makes use of them faster and more efficiently that way. Vitamins at mealtime also help prevent the stomach upsets and diarrhea that some people experience with vitamin supplements.

### Are natural vitamins superior to synthetic vitamins?

Both have the same chemical structures, both have the same biological activity. But synthetic vitamins have this advantage: they're cheaper. However, vitamins A and D derived from fish oils, or B complex vitamins derived from yeast or dried liver, may have an edge in effectiveness over their synthetic counterparts.

### Is it safe to take vitamins in large doses?

Quantities greater than RDAs are regarded by some doctors as worthless in most cases, and sometimes hazardous. However, there is some evidence of the effectiveness of "mega" doses in the treatment of pathological conditions ranging from schizophrenia and hyperactivity in children to cardiovascular diseases and diabetes.

The maximum vitamin potencies on this diet are not even remotely close to established toxicity levels. The toxicity level of vitamin E, for example, is 100,000 IUs; the maximum SDA of vitamin E on this diet is only one tenth of that.

Warning: This diet is meant for adults in consultation with their physicians. It is not meant for children. Vitamins A, D, and E are highly toxic to

# YOUR INDIVIDUAL VITAMIN SDAs (SLIMMING DAILY ALLOWANCES)

| VITAMINS | Your Age: | 19-35 | 36-50 | 50+ |
|---|---|---|---|---|
| A (IU *)<br>(retinol) | | 5,000–10,000 | 5,000–12,000 | 10,000–15,000 |
| D (IU)<br>(cholecalciferol) | | 400–600 | 400–600 | 400–600 |
| E (IU)<br>(alpha tocopherol) | | 100–200 | 200–400 | 400–600 |
| Vitamin C (mg *)<br>(ascorbic acid or calcium or<br>potassium ascorbate) | | 1,000–2,000 | 1,000–3,000 | 2,000–4,000 |
| $B_1$ (mg)<br>(thiamine) | | 50–150 | 100–1500 | 150–200 |
| $B_2$ (mg)<br>(riboflavin) | | 50–150 | 100–150 | 100–200 |
| $B_3$ (mg)<br>(niacin) | | 100–300 | 100–300 | 200–400 |
| $B_6$ (mg)<br>(pyridoxine) | | 50–200 | 100–300 | 200–400 |
| $B_{12}$ (mg)<br>(cobalamine) | | 50–150 | 100–300 | 100–200 |
| Biotin (mcg *)<br>(vitamin H) | | 50–150 | 100–150 | 100–200 |
| Choline † (mg) | | 100–200 | 100–200 | 100–300 |
| Folic acid (mcg)<br>(folacin) | | 500–1,000 | 500–1,000 | 500–1,000 |
| Inositol † (mg) | | 100–200 | 100–200 | 100–300 |
| PABA (mg)<br>(para aminobenzoic acid) | | 50–150 | 50–150 | 100–200 |
| Pantothenic acid | | 100–200 | 100–200 | 100–300 |

* IU stands for International Units, mg for milligrams, mcg for micrograms. There are 454 milligrams in an ounce, and 1,000 micrograms in a milligram.

† Two disputed vitamins, inositol and choline, are included because of the strong evidence of their role in fat metabolism. Two other disputed vitamins, $B_{15}$ and bioflavonoids, are omitted because they appear in sufficient quantity in foods approved for this diet. Vitamin K is also omitted because it is normally manufactured by intestinal flora in the human body.

children in quantities far smaller than those that are toxic in adults. Parents of overweight children could do their offspring serious injury by putting them on this diet.

### Are there any health advantages of SDAs over RDAs?

It is likely that optimal personal allowances of vitamins, on which my SDAs are based, could help ward off subclinical symptoms of vitamin deprivation. These include exhaustion, vague aches and pains, insomnia, headaches, digestive disturbances, poor concentration, palpitations, irritability, and anxiety. These symptoms, however, may arise from other causes as well. SDAs, I believe, have contributed not only to my slimness but to my wellness, both mental and physical.

### If we overeat to obtain enough vitamins to meet the body's demands for peak efficiency, why aren't fat people healthy and vigorous?

We overeat in an *attempt* to obtain enough vitamins to meet the body's demands, but our food is so vitamin impoverished we seldom come close. Most overweights are undernourished, are prone to nutrition-related diseases, and have a shorter life expectancy than most slim people.

### How do I store vitamin supplements?

Keep them in a cool, dark, dry place. Do not refrigerate. Do not discard the absorbent cotton or packets of dessicants supplied by the manufacturer; they absorb moisture and prolong the shelf life of the vitamin product. If no moisture absorbents are included, after opening stuff the empty spaces in the containers with absorbent cotton.

### If vitamins are foods, can't I just live on them?

Absolutely not. They cannot be sub-stituted for proteins, fats, and carbohydrates because they don't do the job of those nutrients, and they don't contribute calories—the energy which makes your body work. It's just plain silly to think you can eat enormous quantities of vitamins and go without other food. It's also dangerous. Use your vitamins *with* food, *never instead of* food.

### Are time-release capsules better for me than regular vitamin supplements?

While it's true that blood levels of vitamin C and B-complex vitamins peak in about 2 hours then decline, it is in the cells of the body not in the blood that the vitamins do their work. Vitamin C and B-complex vitamins taken once a day in sufficient quantities will *probably* ensure the presence of these vitamins in the cells for a 24-hour period. If you don't want to take chances, do use time-release capsules.

Whether you take vitamins as time-release capsules, regular capsules, tablets, liquids, drops, or crystals depends on the answer to these subjective questions: Can you swallow your choice with ease? Can you digest it without discomfort? Can you afford it?

### Do I need mineral supplements while I lose weight?

Yes. Weight loss in the first weeks of this diet is essentially due to the shedding of water (diuresis) because of the dramatic reduction in salt intake. In the opinion of some authorities, that flushing of the system carries away large quantities of water-soluble vitamins (C and members of the B complex) as well as water-soluble minerals (potassium, magnesium, selenium, manganese, copper and so on). The loss of minerals could present an enormous danger. Pharmacological diuretics for the treatment of high blood pressure, weight loss (diet pills), and pre-menstrual bloat have in some cases caused death from potassium depletion. The use of vitamin supplements more than restore the vitamins lost in diuresis; and a mineral supplement that conforms to U.S. RDAs for all minerals should bring back your mineral content to normal. *Normal mineral content is necessary for a normal appestat setting.*

There is a body of research literature which holds that water loss due to salt reduction does not produce the severe effects associated with water loss due to the use of pharmacological diuretics. But it is wise to take the stand of a nutritional conservative; if there is even the slightest hint of danger, protect yourself against it. The mineral supplements recommended here can be obtained wherever vitamins are sold; and many vitamin supplements also contain minerals. Chelated minerals are preferred, since they pass through cell membranes more readily than unchelated ones, and help provide your body with the mineral concentrations you intend it to have. Read labels.

### Do I need mineral supplements on a maintenance diet?

According to the U.S. Department of Agriculture, it is virtually impossible to design a diet of whole, fresh, and unprocessed foods (no less pre-cooked, prepared, and packaged foods) of less than 2,000 calories a day that provides even U.S. RDA quantities of all minerals. Dr. Mark O. Hegsted of the U.S. Department of Agriculture notes that "most women between 23 and 55, and many men, consume [only] 1,500 calories a day on the average." If you weigh less than 135 pounds, you probably are consuming less than 2,000 calories a day, and a supplement that conforms to U.S. RDAs for all minerals should be part of your diet, provided your physician approves.*

### I've heard that excess minerals are dangerous. Is that true?

Excess minerals can build up in your body, and when they reach a critical amount, they can turn poisonous and sometimes toxic. It is prudent to consume no more than the U.S. RDAs for minerals. And, as with vitamin supplements, never add mineral supplements to your diet without consulting your doctor.

---

* On the other hand, Dr. Hegsted interprets his data as meaning "the RDAs have been set too high, rather than that most women are suffering from deficiency."

CHAPTER

# 16

# EXERCISE: IT LETS YOU
# CHEAT HEALTHFULLY OR
# LOSE WEIGHT FASTER

Yes, you *can* cheat. What's even more wonderful, you can cheat while dropping pounds *and* improving your figure.

The secret is exercise.

Exercise replaces flabby fat with lean protein that occupies only a fraction of the volume of fat tissue. You lose inches where you need to lose them most. You look trimmer, fitter, more attractive than sedentary people of the same weight. In combination with this diet, exercise slims you down while it shapes you up. Exercise, states Nathan Pritikin, has "a rapid beautifying effect" on the dieter.

But exercise also burns off calories. That means, if your diet calls for X calories, and you burn off, say, 20 percent of X calories with exercise, then you can add 20 percent of X calories to your diet—*and still lose weight*. Why not, then, add cheat foods to your diet—like ice cream, malted milkshakes, pizzas, strawberry shortcake, candy bars—then burn them off with exercise?

"Great!" respond some dieters to whom cheating is a necessity. It helps them get through the take-it-off days,

and eases the transition to a stay-thin diet. If you're one of those dieters, by all means cheat. But cheat *my* way. Enjoy that malted milkshake, then run for 46 minutes, or jog for 63 minutes, or golf for 100 minutes to burn it off. Be sure you exercise away every no-no you put away.

How much exercise do you need to cheat? That depends on what you're cheating on, and what kind of exercise you're going on. The chart on the following page takes both factors into account and gives you the right numbers. You won't find on it all the foods you should forget but can't; there's no peach pie on it, for example, but you will find apple pie, and the numbers are much the same. When you can't find what you're looking for, look for something like it. Numbers are ball park, so err on the side of too much exercise rather than too little.

But if you don't cheat, exercise can melt off extra pounds while you're dieting. The chart on page 85 will tell you how many hours of your favorite exercises you need to lose a pound.

83

# A CHEATER'S GUIDE TO EXERCISING IT OFF

To cheat with these foods . . .    . . . exercise with the activity of your choice for the number of minutes listed.

| | WALKING | JOGGING | RUNNING | CYCLING | SWIMMING | TENNIS | GOLF | SKATING | BOWLING | HOUSEWORK |
|---|---|---|---|---|---|---|---|---|---|---|
| Bacon and eggs | 60 | 44 | 32 | 50 | 44 | 44 | 70 | 50 | 70 | 70 |
| Doughnut | 25 | 19 | 14 | 15 | 19 | 19 | 30 | 22 | 30 | 30 |
| Pancakes with syrup | 140 | 105 | 76 | 84 | 205 | 105 | 168 | 120 | 168 | 168 |
| Delicatessen club sandwich | 98 | 74 | 54 | 59 | 74 | 74 | 118 | 84 | 118 | 118 |
| Spaghetti with sauce | 66 | 50 | 36 | 40 | 50 | 50 | 80 | 57 | 80 | 80 |
| Pizza (slice) | 30 | 23 | 16 | 18 | 23 | 23 | 36 | 26 | 36 | 36 |
| Chicken TV dinner | 57 | 48 | 31 | 34 | 43 | 43 | 69 | 49 | 69 | 67 |
| Southern fried chicken | 77 | 58 | 42 | 46 | 58 | 58 | 92 | 66 | 92 | 92 |
| Chocolate chip cookies (6) | 51 | 38 | 28 | 31 | 38 | 38 | 68 | 44 | 61 | 61 |
| Ice cream (scoop) | 32 | 24 | 17 | 19 | 24 | 24 | 39 | 28 | 39 | 39 |
| Ice cream soda | 43 | 32 | 23 | 26 | 32 | 32 | 51 | 36 | 51 | 51 |
| Malted milkshake | 84 | 63 | 46 | 50 | 63 | 63 | 100 | 72 | 100 | 100 |
| Layer cake (slice) | 60 | 44 | 32 | 50 | 44 | 44 | 70 | 50 | 70 | 70 |
| Apple pie (slice) | 63 | 47 | 34 | 38 | 47 | 47 | 75 | 54 | 75 | 75 |
| Baked custard | 25 | 19 | 14 | 15 | 19 | 19 | 30 | 21 | 30 | 30 |
| Eclair | 48 | 36 | 26 | 29 | 36 | 36 | 58 | 41 | 58 | 58 |
| Strawberry shortcake | 67 | 50 | 36 | 40 | 50 | 50 | 80 | 57 | 80 | 80 |
| Candy bar | 50 | 38 | 27 | 30 | 38 | 38 | 60 | 43 | 60 | 60 |

# HOW MUCH EXERCISE YOU NEED TO
# LOSE ONE POUND

| Exercise | Hours |
|---|---|
| Badminton | 10 |
| Ballet exercises | 10 |
| Bowling | 12 |
| Calisthenics | 10 |
| Cycling (6 miles an hour) | 12 |
| (8 miles an hour) | 10 |
| (10 miles an hour) | 8 |
| (11 miles an hour) | 7 |
| (12 miles an hour) | 6 |
| (13 miles an hour) | 5 |
| Dancing (ballroom) | 12 |
| (disco) | 4 |
| Downhill skiing | 6 |
| Golf (carrying clubs) | 10 |
| (pulling cart) | 12 |
| (with power cart) | 15 |
| Handball (light workout) | 5 |
| Housework (heavy) | 12 |
| (light) | 23 |
| Jogging (5 miles an hour) | 6 |
| Paddle ball | 6 |
| Running (5.5 miles an hour) | 5 |
| (6 to 8 miles an hour) | 4 |
| Skating (ice or roller) | 8 |
| Squash (light workout) | 5 |
| Table tennis | 10 |
| Tennis (doubles) | 10 |
| (singles) | 7 |
| Volleyball | 10 |
| Walking (1 mile in an hour) | 23 |
| (2 to 3 miles in an hour) | 12 |
| (3.5 miles in an hour) | 10 |
| (4 miles in an hour) | 8 |
| (5 miles in an hour) | 7 |
| Water skiing | 7 |

Note: You'll need about 10 percent less exercise time if you're under 150 pounds, and about 10 percent more if you're over.

# EXERCISE CAN MAKE YOU FEEL BETTER—MENTALLY AND PHYSICALLY

The best kind of exercise involves the whole body, particularly the legs, because that kind of exercise causes the blood (and the oxygen it carries) to course to every part of the body. Your heart doesn't have to work so hard, each of your cells glows with vitality, and you even think faster and better.

Exercise, asserts weight-control expert Dr. Joseph Rechtshaffen, "reduces risk of heart disease . . . helps relieve arthritis and diabetes . . . promotes longevity," and even "motivates you to stop smoking."

Dr. Jeremiah Stamler, the eminent nutritionist, adds, "Exercise may help keep blood pressure under control. [It] may slow down changes that occur with aging—stiffness . . . and loss of muscle tone. You are likely to sleep better. And be much better able to undertake a sudden run for a bus or train . . . without harm."

Exercise, combined with a healthful diet, gives you the capacity to live your life to the fullest.

"But," I'm often asked, "there are so many kinds of exercise—aerobics, isotonics, calisthenics. . . . What kind of exercise is right for me?"

"Whatever one involves your whole body and gives you the most pleasure," I answer. "But I recommend—"

# THE EXERCISE FOR EVERYBODY: WALKING

When Dr. Norman Jolliffe tested his Prudent Diet on 1,100 human guinea pigs, he insisted that each of them walk several miles a day. The experiment wasn't only a smashing weight-reducing success, but it also cut the rate of heart attack by an unprecedented 500 percent and helped ward off or normalize a long list of maladies. Walking is healthful.

It's also an exercise that requires no training, equipment, uniform, or membership fee. It's natural and it's free. You just get out there and walk. When I do, a splendid thing happens. Other exercises fatigue me; but this exercise walks tiredness away. After a few-miles hike at three miles an hour, I return to my kitchen or typewriter eager to get going. I feel I can go on for hours and hours and hours, and I do.

So many medically backed claims have been made for walking that I could write a book about them. But, in a capsule: Walking is nature's tranquilizer. It's a disposition changer (for the better). It can help depress cholesterol levels, prevent heart attack. It fights bone shrinkage, the scourge of many aging women. It eases headache pains. It helps restore vigor and well-being after illness. And it's safe.

You don't have to be an exercise nut to benefit from exercise. You can walk.

# PRACTICAL TIPS ON HOW TO GET THE MOST FROM EXERCISE

*I've never really exercised. What's my first step?*

Tell your doctor you're planning an exercise program. He or she will give you a complete physical, including a stress test (to see how your heart reacts to exercise), plus advice on how to go about exercising without risk.

*What's better for me—walking or jogging?*

You lose weight faster jogging, but not much faster than by walking rapidly. Your circulatory system gets a better workout when jogging than when walking, and that's a point in jogging's favor. But joggers have come down with a number of leg ailments unknown to walkers, and that's a point against it. If jogging is fun for you, stick to it. But if it isn't, and I must confess I've never seen a happy-looking jogger—then try the unqualified joys of walking.

*I can only get to the tennis court on weekends. Okay?*

Not okay. You have to exercise consistently to benefit from it. Why don't you start walking on weekdays—before breakfast or after dinner are great times—and fill out your exercise week with tennis on weekends?

*I like walking and I like jogging. But when the weather's bad I can't do either. Suggestion?*

Jog in place at home.

*Can I use a home exercise bicycle or a cross-country machine?*

Yes. Or you can save money by learning how to skip rope.

*What's wrong with working out at a Y or health club?*

Nothing, as long as you exercise consistently. Walk on the days you can't work out.

*Are isotonic exercises and weight-lifting good for me?*

They're exercises for developing particular muscles. They're not as helpful to you as exercises involving all parts of the body.

*What are aerobics? And can I benefit from them?*

Aerobics are strenuous exercises developed in the 1960s for the Air Force by Dr. Kenneth Cooper. "Aerobics," states Dr. Edward B. Diethrich, director of the Arizona Heart Institute, "are the best type of exercise for weight control. . . . After several months of training . . . the muscles you use will begin to firm up and the weight you lose will be distributed over your entire body." Aerobic exercise dances are not quite as strenuous as the original Air Force exercises, and look like much more fun.

*I've been told that if I exercise before meals I'll lose weight faster. True or false?*

True, because you'll lose some of your appetite. In general, according to weight-control expert Dr. Joseph Rechtshaffen, exercise "decreases appetite [and] helps promote weight loss." Dr. Jeremiah Stamler, chairman of the Department of Community Health and Preventive Medicine, Northwestern University Medical School, added that "many people . . . tend to eat *less* once they become physically fit." (Emphasis his.)

*I've been told I should warm up before exercise and cool down after exercise. How do I do that?*

You can warm up and cool down with stretch exercises. Write for *Everyday Stretch*, a complete guide to stretching, P.O. Box 767, Palmer Lake, Colorado 80133.

*Salt is virtually taboo on your diet. But what about salt tablets?*

Check with your doctor. You may be told that even when you exercise hard in hot weather, some salt on your food is all that's necessary.

*After strenuous exercises, I know I lose fluids and also sodium and potassium. I have to replace them, right? What about Gatorade?*

Fine, as far as it goes. But Dr. Patricia Beckwith of Children's Hospital in Los Angeles reports a drawback. Gatorade and other fluid replacement drinks are so concentrated with minerals that they can't be absorbed directly. Water must be drawn to the stomach from other parts of the body. This takes time, and the effect of the drink is delayed. For quick action Dr. Beckwith suggests diluting your Gatorade, or similar drink, with water before swallowing.

# 17

## GETTING IT OFF
## AFTER YOU'VE PUT IT BACK ON

What dieter who has reached desired weight hasn't come back bulging with extra pounds from a weekend with friends, a wedding, a vacation, holidays with the folks, a convention, or even a night on the town?

It's human.

There are times when it's good for your spirits to let yourself go.

Don't feel guilty.

Don't wallow in remorse.

And, above all, don't feel you're climbing up the yo-yo again.

You *won't* when you take action immediately to—

## DROP 5 TO 7 POUNDS A WEEK WITHOUT GIVING UP A SINGLE CALORIE

All you have to do is go back on your Thin-for-Life Program, which you would have done anyway. You'll lose some or all of the weight you regained while you enjoy three major meals and four satisfying snacks a day.

*That sounds impossible. You'll have to explain that to me.*

Gladly. Once you're down to weight on this no-salt diet, your biggest enemy is not overeating, but eating too much salt. The rule of thumb is: For every 1,000 milligrams of sodium consumed over 400 milligrams, you retain two pounds of water. (Sodium is the main constituent of salt.) Most Americans consume about 4,000 to 5,000 milli-

grams of sodium a day (equivalent to a bit more than one and a half teaspoons of salt). When you put back weight by returning to the average American diet, you could regain as much as seven to nine pounds in water weight alone.

When you go back on my salt-free Thin-for-Life Program, you'll lose water at the rate of at least four pounds a week. The amazing weight loss on The One-Week Crash Diet is due in large part to water loss induced by low salt intake. "There are many reports of 10 to 12 or more pounds of weight lost through water excretion in the first week of dieting," Dr. Jolliffe wrote. "Five to seven pounds in the first week is not uncommon."

89

*How do I know when I've lost all my
excess water?*
When your bathroom scale shows no
further weight loss for three consecutive
days.

*What shall I do after I've lost all my
excess water and I'm still a few pounds
overweight?*
Go back on the One-Week Crash Diet.
You'll have no trouble taking it off at
the rate of 2 to 2½ pounds a week.
  Any other questions?

*Yes. If a normal appestat holds my food
intake to normal, how come I overeat on
vacations?*

You eat the wrong kinds of foods—foods
heavy in salt, sugar, and excess fat.
They're appetite stimulants that reset
the appestat too high. You also probably forget to take your vitamins.

  Salt is your major enemy. It's hidden
in almost everything you eat out—and in
great quantities. Just as you lose water
weight when you cut down on salt, so
you gain it when you increase your salt
intake.

*I've got a toughie. I do everything you
say on your Thin-for-Life Program, yet I
gain weight. How come?*
The answer is, you're playing—

# THE DIETER'S MOST DANGEROUS GAME: "INVISIBLE EATING"

"Do you eat more than you should?" I
asked the questioner.
  "No."
  "Sure?"
  "Positive. I eat like a bird."
  "Why don't you do this?" I said. "It's
an experiment. Get yourself a small pad
and pencil. Carry it around with you—at
home, in the office, every place. Jot
down everything you eat that's *not* on
the diet. *Everything.* No matter how
small."
  "No matter how small? One peanut?"
  "Half a peanut."
  A few days later she came back to me
with a neat list headed *Extras for the
Day.* It included "a half-slice bread . . . 6
cashew nuts [this was repeated many
times] . . . dabs of mayonnaise . . . a
spoonful of ice cream . . . 4 jelly beans
. . . a sixth of a slice of chocolate layer
cake . . . half a peanut . . ." It was a long
list.
  "But they're such small amounts," she

said. "How many calories can they add
up to?"
  I made the calculations.
  "About three hundred."
  "About *three hundred!* I didn't real-
ize I was eating *anything.*"
  That's "invisible eating"—a game of
self-deception. It's played with quantities of food so small they're out of
your mind before they're out of your
mouth. In this case, the game accounted
for a weight gain of about half a pound
a week. (She consumed 2,100 extra calories a week. It takes an extra 3,500 to
put on a pound.) She said she ate like a
bird. Of course she did. Birds nibble all
day. So did she.

*How do I break my "invisible eating"
habit?*
Easily. Carry around a pad and pencil.
Then before you reach for an "extra,"
jot down what you're *going to* eat. Now
that you're very conscious of your food,

it's no longer "invisible." Chances are you won't eat it.

After a while you won't need the pad and pencil. You'll have formed a new eating habit: you'll reject nibbles automatically. You'll no longer eat like a bird; you'll eat like a human being.

# 18

# THE BIG BONUS:
# A HEALTHIER YOU

Dr. Myron Winick, director of the Institute of Human Nutrition at Columbia University in New York, in a recent statement to the press stated that half of all Americans are malnourished—most because they eat too much, and some because they don't eat enough of the *right foods* (my emphasis).

He said that Americans eat the wrong kinds of food, particularly those containing too much saturated fat, which has been linked to heart disease, and too much salt, which can be a factor in high blood pressure (hypertension).

"Bad nutrition involving both excessive nutrient intake and nutrient deficiencies is unnecessarily shortening the life span of millions of Americans," he concluded.

## THIS APPETITE-CONTROL DIET CONTAINS THE *RIGHT FOODS* AND HAS NO NUTRIENT DEFICIENCIES

The Vitamin Diet is low in saturated fat, and is low in salt. It is also low in fat and cholesterol, and permits little sugar. All these nutrients have been indicted by modern medical science as potentially harmful. This diet has no nutrient deficiencies; it is high in fiber and is supplemented with RDAs of minerals and optimal quantities of vitamins. It also helps prevent overeating by controlling the weight-regulating mechanism at the base of the brain, the appestat.

This diet conforms more closely than any other popular diet to the nutritional guidelines set by the U.S. Department of Agriculture, the U.S. Department of Human Services, and those set by Dr. Norman Jolliffe for the Bureau of Nutrition, New York City Department of Health. It is an improvement over the average American diet in the following ways:

• *This diet lowers fat consumption.* Low fat fights obesity, heart attack, diabetes, and other nutrition-related diseases and reduces the risk of cancer. Excess fat is an appetite stimulant. The amount of fat on this diet is about 20 percent in terms of total calories; on the average American diet, about 45 percent.

• *This diet raises the ratio of polyun-*

*saturated fat to saturated fat.* Poly-unsaturated fats are regarded by many medical researchers as essentially healthful, and saturated fats as potentially harmful. The ratio of polyunsaturated fats to saturated fats on this diet is about 4 to 1; on the average American diet, about 0.2 to 1.

• *This diet reduces cholesterol consumption.* "Individuals . . . with diets high in cholesterol," the *Federal Dietary Guidelines for Americans* asserts, "usually have greater risk of heart attacks than people eating . . . low-cholesterol diets." Cholesterol intake on this diet is about 160 to 185 milligrams a day; on the average American diet, 720.

• *This diet increases the consumption of complex carbohydrates.* "Complex carbohydrate foods are better than simple carbohydrate foods in this regard. Simple carbohydrates—such as sugars—provide calories but little else in the way of nutrients. Complex carbohydrate foods—such as beans, peas, nuts, seeds, fruits and vegetables, and whole-grain breads, cereals, and products—contain many essential nutrients in addition to calories" (*Federal Dietary Guidelines for Americans*). This diet in terms of total calories is about 60 percent carbohydrate, mostly complex; the average American diet is about 50 percent carbohydrate, mostly simple.

• *This diet steps up protein consumption.* Dr. Norman Jolliffe wrote: "Without an adequate amount of high-value protein in each meal, the reducer may develop weakness, nervousness, increased fatigability, and other symptoms of protein deficiency." This diet contains about 20 percent protein in terms of total calories; the average American diet, about 10 to 15 percent.

• *This diet boosts fiber content.* The *Federal Dietary Guidelines for Americans* states: "Eating more foods high in fiber tends to reduce the symp-toms of chronic constipation, diverticulosis, and some types of 'irritable bowel.' There is also concern that low-fiber diets might increase the risks of developing cancer of the colon." Dr. Joseph Rechtshaffen adds that a high-fiber diet "reduces risk of hemorrhoids, varicose veins, hiatus hernia, phlebitis, and gall bladder disease . . . prevents both constipation and diarrhea . . . lowers absorption of fats, thereby lowering blood cholesterol . . . [and] reduces risk of heart disease." This diet contains about 15 grams or more of fiber per day; the average American diet, less than 5 grams.

• *This diet minimizes sugar (sucrose).* "The major hazard from eating too much sugar," states the *Federal Dietary Guidelines for Americans*, "is tooth decay (dental caries)." Sucrose has been associated by many medical investigators with heart attack and other degenerative diseases. Sugar is an appetite stimulant, and an empty calorie. On this diet there is no added sugar (there is some naturally occurring sucrose); about 18 percent of the average American diet is composed of sugar.

• *This diet minimizes salt.* Marion Burros, the nutrition expert, wrote: "Some 40 million to 60 million Americans suffer from hypertension, with more than 40 percent of the population over 65 afflicted. It has been called the silent killer because it often has no outward symptoms until heart disease, stroke, or kidney failure have taken their toll. The medical community is almost unanimous in its belief that there is a link between hypertension and the consumption of sodium." Sodium is the major constituent of salt.

In addition to reducing the risk of hypertension, a "low-salt diet," according to Dr. Joseph Rechtshaffen, "reduces edema (fluid retention in the body) . . . premenstrual bloating and tension . . .

[and] promotes weight loss." This diet contains about 500 to 2,000 milligrams of sodium per day; the average American diet, 4,500 to 5,000.

• *This diet supplies U.S. RDAs of minerals.* "The best way to get your daily requirements of essential minerals [macrominerals and trace minerals]," advises an eminent nutritionist, "is through the foods you eat. Except for iron and possibly zinc, a reasonably well-structured diet will give your body what it needs for good health without destroying the proper balance and amounts of various minerals."

This is true, according to the Department of Agriculture, on diets in excess of 2,000 calories a day. But on cooking, essential water-soluble minerals are often left in the pot. So even on over-2,000-calorie-a-day diets, mineral supplements are necessary. This diet makes use of supplements conforming to the RDAs of *all* minerals for its reducing and maintenance programs. It also em-

ploys optimal supplementary quantities of Vitamin C, which aids in the absorption of iron. The average American diet below 2,000 calories is likely to be deficient in most or all minerals; and at higher calorie levels may at some times be deficient in iron, magnesium, zinc, and calcium. Its vitamin C levels are frequently too low to help appreciably in the absorption of iron.

• *This diet is supplemented with optimal quantities of vitamins.* "Supplementation," asserts vitamin expert Robert J. Benowicz, "can support and reinforce good health practices [such as] appropriate exercise and an intelligent diet. [But] relying on vitamins alone for good health is absurd. [They] cannot bestow immunity on a body that continues to be metabolically maltreated and physically abused." On this diet, vitamin supplements are integrated into a comprehensive diet and exercise program. They are not in average American life.

## HOW THE VITAMIN DIET
## COMPARES TO THE AVERAGE AMERICAN DIET

| Nutrients | Average Diet | The Vitamin Diet |
|---|---|---|
| Fat * <br> The lower the better | 40–45 | 20 |
| P:S (ratio of polyunsaturated fat to saturated fat) <br> The higher the better | 0.2:1 | 4:1 |
| Cholesterol † <br> 160–85 is prudent | 720 | 160–85 |
| Carbohydrates * <br> 50–65 is prudent; <br> Complex is better than simple | 40–50 <br> mostly simple | 60 <br> mostly complex |
| Protein * <br> 15–20 is prudent | 10–15 | 20 |
| Fiber ‡ <br> 15 or more is prudent | 5 | 15+ |
| Sugar (sucrose) * <br> The lower the better | 16 | little added |
| Sodium <br> About 275 mgs a day is all the body needs | 4,000–5,000 | 500–2,000 |
| Minerals <br> U.S. RDAs are sufficient | U.S. RDAs | U.S. RDAs |
| Vitamins <br> Optimal is better | Minimal | Optimal |

* Percent of total calories
† Milligrams
‡ Grams

## WHAT VITAMIN SUPPLEMENTS CAN DO FOR YOU AS PART OF A TOTAL DIET AND EXERCISE PROGRAM

In general, vitamin supplements can help—

- Improve general health
- Fight infections and degenerative diseases
- Hold back the aging clock
- Lengthen the life span
- Counter the effects of excessive use of alcohol and nicotine
- Alleviate fatigue
- Correct past nutritional abuses
- Relieve stress (personal and environmental)
- Keep the body operating at peak efficiency

# SPECIFIC VITAMINS
# CAN BOOST THE HEALTH
# OF THE PARTS AND FUNCTIONS
# OF THE BODY

| Part or Function | Vitamins |
| --- | --- |
| Blood | $B_1$, $B_2$, $B_6$, $B_{12}$, biotin, E, folic acid, K, PABA |
| Bones | A, C, D, K |
| Carbohydrate metabolism | $B_1$, pantothenic acid |
| Cardiovascular system | $B_1$, $B_3$, C, choline, E, inositol |
| Cartilage | C |
| Circulatory system | E |
| Collagen | C |
| Digestion of polyunsaturated fats | E |
| Energy production | $B_1$, $B_2$, $B_3$, biotin |
| Eyes | A, $B_1$, $B_2$, $B_3$, C, D, K |
| Fat metabolism | $B_6$, biotin, C, choline, inositol, pantothenic acid |
| Hair | A, biotin |
| Immune system | C |
| Intestines | $B_1$, $B_3$, $B_6$ |
| Iron absorption | C |
| Mucus membranes | A, $B_2$ |
| Muscles | E |
| Nervous system | $B_1$, $B_3$, $B_6$, $B_{12}$, folic acid, choline, pantothenic acid |
| Protein metabolism | A, $B_6$, C, pantothenic acid |
| Repair mechanism | $B_1$ |
| Reproduction | A, $B_{12}$, E, folic acid |
| Skin | A, $B_2$, $B_3$, $B_6$, biotin, C, K |
| Teeth development | A, $B_6$, C, D |
| Wound healing | C, K |

Specific vitamins also combat the common cold (C), menopausal distress (E), and leg cramps (E, C, D, and K). Vitamins A, C, E, and pantothenic acid may help prevent cancer. Stress is fought by vitamins A, $B_6$, E, and pantothenic acid; and vitamins A, C, E, and pantothenic acid combat environmental pollution. $B_3$ may help migraine; $B_{12}$, generalized aches and pains; and C, $B_1$, $B_3$, E, and possibly $B_{15}$, heart disease. D seems to be helpful against lead and other metal poisonings. C and E may be the youth vitamins that help keep you feeling and looking younger longer.

# WOMEN'S NUTRITIONAL PROBLEMS: HOW THIS DIET HELPS SOLVE SOME OF THEM

"Nutrient deficiencies in this country's adults are . . . a problem for women because of lifestyle and life-change problems—menstruation, pregnancy, breastfeeding, and the pill," Dr. Myron Winick observed. "The major deficiencies are generally in iron, calcium, folic acid, and vitamin $B_6$, and lead to anemia and brittle bones."

If you're a woman, the first step in treating nutrient deficiencies is a visit to your physician. You may be told that a diet such as my maintenance diet can be helpful. It is naturally rich in iron and calcium, contains optimal amounts of vitamins C and D, which aid in the metabolism of these elements, and also contains folic acid in optimal amounts.

# CALORIE AND SODIUM CONTENTS OF THE VITAMIN DIET

Low calorie intake means less fat weight; low sodium intake means less water weight.

When directions are followed by the average American explicitly (salad *must* be eaten before the entrée, for example), the Crash Diet contributes about 1,200 to 1,600 calories a day, and up to 2,000 milligrams of sodium. Each Binge Day contributes about 1,600 to 2,000 calories a day, plus up to 2,000 milligrams of sodium. The Thin-for-Life maintenance diet contributes enough calories to maintain your ideal weight, and 500 to 2,000 milligrams of sodium.

Remember, how much *you* eat is determined by your appestat, and *your* calorie counts on the crash and binge weeks are likely to vary from the average figures I've given.

This, then, is the Vitamin Diet. More than a diet for weight loss and weight control, it's a lifetime program for healthful living. It's a program designed with tender loving care for you and for all for whom you care. It's a program for food lovers everywhere. It's a program that exalts the joys of being alive—with a serene mind in a happy body.

# The Vitamin Diet Gourmet Mini-Cookbook

*Delicious low-calorie, low-fat, low-saturated-fat, low-cholesterol, high-fiber cooking and baking recipes using no sugar or salt!*

# CONTENTS

# 1

# YES-YES FOODS FOR SLIMNESS AND HEALTH

The foods listed here do not exhaust the possibilities for slim and healthful eating. There are, for example, about 500 varieties of fish and shellfish available in this country, and I include only about 55. But where would you find dogfish, lizard fish, hogsuckers, gags, grunts, croakers, viperfish, brown bullheads, ratfish, roachfish, and white crappies—even if you would want to? (Despite their names, though, they're quite palatable, the U.S. Marine Fisheries Service assures us.)

The foods on my approved list are obtainable for the most part in supermarkets. The few foods you can buy more readily in health food stores are indicated by an asterisk. While you don't have to count calories or sodium content on this diet (I've done both for you), you may be interested to know just how many calories and how much sodium are in common units or measures of these healthful foods. You'll find those figures here. Remember, it's too many calories that put excess fat weight on you, and too much sodium that bloats you with excess water weight.

# HAUTE CUISINE OF HEALTH FOODS *

| Food | Unit or Measure | Calories | Sodium† |
|------|------|------|------|
| *Beverages* | | | |
| Apple cider | ½ cup | 62 | 1 |
| Apple juice | ½ cup | 62 | 6 |
| Apricot juice | ½ cup | 51 | 4 |
| Cranberry juice (unsweetened) | ½ cup | 90 | 3 |
| Coffee | | | |
| Imitation (no caffeine) | 1 TB | 7 | 1 |
| Decaffeinated, instant | 1 TB | 0 | 1 |
| Grape juice | ½ cup | 85 | 4 |
| Grapefruit juice | ½ cup | 65 | 2 |
| Lemon juice | ½ cup | 32 | 2 |
| Orange juice | ½ cup | 34 | 3 |
| Pineapple juice | ½ cup | 60 | 3 |
| Prune juice | ½ cup | 85 | 2 |
| | | | |
| *Breads and Crackers* | | | |
| Crackers | | | |
| Brown rice wafers | 1 | 9 | 1 |
| Wheat wafers | 1 | 8 | 1 |
| Haute cuisine of health breads | slice | 51 | 2 |
| Matzohs (Passover) | 1 | 112 | 0 |
| Melba toast (commercial low-sodium) | 1 | 15 | 2 |
| | | | |
| *Eggs and Dairy Products* | | | |
| Buttermilk (no salt added) | 1 cup | 89 | 120 |
| Cheese | | | |
| Cottage cheese (dry curd, skim milk, less than ½% milkfat, no salt added) | 1 cup | 12 | 42 |
| Low-fat | ½ oz. | 42–100 | 25–50 |
| Eggs | | | |
| Whole | 1 | 87 | 68 |
| Yolk | 1 | 61 | 13 |
| White | 1 | 26 | 55 |
| Milk | | | |
| Evaporated skim | ½ cup | 90 | 128 |
| Nonfat (dry) | 1 TB | 30 | 43 |
| Nonfat (liquid) | 1 cup | 90 | 128 |
| Yogurt (low-fat plain) | 1 cup | 115 | 129 |

*
†  See footnote on page 109.
‡

| Food | Unit or Measure | Calories | Sodium† | |
|------|-----------------|----------|---------|---|
| *Fish* | | | | |
| Abalone | 4 oz. | 125 | 80 | (E)‡ |
| Barracuda | 4 oz. | 129 | 80 | (E) |
| Bass | | | | |
|   Sea | 4 oz. | 110 | 78 | |
|   Small- or large-mouth | 4 oz. | 119 | 80 | (E) |
|   Striped | 4 oz. | 120 | 80 | (E) |
|   White | 4 oz. | 112 | 80 | (E) |
| Bluefish | 4 oz. | 135 | 85 | |
| Butterfish | 4 oz. | 183 | 80 | |
| Carp | 4 oz. | 132 | 57 | |
| Catfish | 4 oz. | 118 | 69 | |
| Clams (meat only) | 4 oz. | 87 | 123 | |
| Cod | 4 oz. | 89 | 80 | |
| Crab | 4 oz. | 160 | 100 | (E) |
| Crayfish | 4 oz. | 82 | 100 | (E) |
| Flounder | 4 oz. | 93 | 89 | |
| Frog's legs | 4 oz. | 83 | 80 | (E) |
| Haddock | 4 oz. | 90 | 70 | |
| Halibut | 4 oz. | 144 | 60 | |
| Herring | | | | |
|   Atlantic | 4 oz. | 210 | 74 | |
|   Pacific | 4 oz. | 112 | 85 | |
| Lobster | 4 oz. | 82 | 100 | |
| Mackerel | 4 oz. | 182 | 60 | |
| Mullet | 4 oz. | 167 | 93 | |
| Mussels (meat only) | 4 oz. | 109 | 320 | |
| Oysters (meat only) | 4 oz. | 80 | 84 | |
| Perch | | | | |
|   White or yellow | 4 oz. | 134 | 80 | |
|   Ocean (redfish) | 4 oz. | 106 | 77 | |
| Pike | 4 oz. | 106 | 58 | |
| Pollack | 4 oz. | 109 | 55 | |
| Porgy | 4 oz. | 129 | 72 | |
| Redfish (ocean perch) | 4 oz. | 106 | 77 | |
| Rockfish | 4 oz. | 113 | 68 | |
| Salmon | | | | |
|   Canned (in water, no salt added) | 4 oz. | 221 | 95 | |
|   Fresh, Atlantic | 4 oz. | 248 | 80 | (E) |
|   Fresh, pink (humpback) | 4 oz. | 136 | 73 | |
| Scallops | 4 oz. | 90 | 85 | (E) |
| Scrod | 4 oz. | 93 | 89 | |
| Sea bass | 4 oz. | 119 | 80 | (E) |
| Shad | 4 oz. | 195 | 62 | |
| Shrimp | 4 oz. | 104 | 159 | |

| Food | Unit or Measure | Calories | Sodium† | |
|------|-----------------|----------|---------|---|
| Skate | 4 oz. | 110 | 80 | (E) |
| Smelts | 4 oz. | 131 | 80 | (E) |
| Snails | 4 oz. | 103 | 80 | (E) |
| Snapper | 4 oz. | 106 | 74 | |
| Squid | 4 oz. | 95 | 80 | (E) |
| Sturgeon | 4 oz. | 167 | 80 | (E) |
| Swordfish | 4 oz. | 140 | 90 | |
| Tilefish | 4 oz. | 92 | 80 | (E) |
| Trout | | | | |
|    Brook | 4 oz. | 115 | 80 | |
|    Lake | 4 oz. | 160 | 80 | |
| Tuna | | | | |
|    Canned (in water, no salt added) | 4 oz. | 122 | 60 | |
|    Fresh, bluefin | 4 oz. | 167 | 45 | |
|    Fresh, yellowfin | 4 oz. | 108 | 86 | |
| | | | | |
| *Flours and Yeast* | | | | |
| All-purpose (unbleached enriched) | ¼ cup | 104 | 0 | |
| Buckwheat | ¼ cup | 88 | 0 | |
| Corn | ¼ cup | 102 | 3 | |
| Gluten | ¼ cup | 108 | 0 | |
| Pastry | ¼ cup | 104 | 0 | |
| Rye (medium) | ¼ cup | 100 | 0 | |
| Wheat (whole) | ¼ cup | 100 | 3 | |
| Soybean (defatted) | ¼ cup | 63 | 0 | |
| Yeast (granular) | 1 TB | 20 | 0 | |
| | | | | |
| *Fruit* | | | | |
| Apples | 1 med. | 75 | 4 | |
| Apricots | 1 med. | 18 | 1 | |
|    Dried | 1 med. | 20 | 2 | |
| Bananas | 1 med. | 99 | 6 | |
| Blackberries | ¼ cup | 18 | 12 | |
| Blueberries | ¼ cup | 21 | 1 | |
| Cantaloupe | ¼ med. | 18 | 6 | |
| Casaba melon | 1 med. wedge | 27 | 12 | |
| Cherries | ¼ cup | 20 | 2 | |
| Crabapples | 1 avg. | 20 | 1 | |
| Cranberries | ¼ cup | 14 | 1 | |
| Currants | ¼ cup | 15 | 1 | |
| Dates (dried) | 1 avg. | 22 | 0 | |
| Date sugar (powder) | 1 TB | 60 | 1 | (E) |
| Figs | 1 avg. | 40 | 1 | |
|    Dried | 1 avg. | 77 | 3 | |
| Gooseberries | ¼ cup | 15 | 0 | |

| Food | Unit or Measure | Calories | Sodium† |
|---|---|---|---|
| Grapefruit | ½ med. | 75 | 3 |
| Grapes | 1 med. | 5 | 0 |
| Guava | 1 avg. | 50 | 2 |
| Honeydew melon | 1 med. wedge | 33 | 12 |
| Huckleberries | ½ cup | 80 | 1 |
| Lemons | 1 med. | 20 | 0 |
| Limes | 1 med. | 20 | 0 |
| Loganberries | ¼ cup | 23 | 0 |
| Mangoes | 1 med. | 133 | 0 |
| Nectarines | 1 med. | 40 | 4 |
| Oranges | 1 med. | 70 | 2 |
| Papayas | 1 med. | 43 | 6 |
| Peaches | 1 avg. | 51 | 2 |
| Pears | 1 avg. | 60 | 2 |
| Persimmons | 1 avg. | 95 | 9 |
| Pineapples | | | |
|   Canned (in its own juice) | | | |
|   Cubes | ¼ cup | 19 | 0 |
|   Fresh | ¼-in. slice | 35 | 0 |
| Plums | 1 avg. | 29 | 0 |
| Pomegranate | 1 avg. | 75 | 3 |
| Prunes | 1 avg. | 16 | 3 |
| Pumpkin | ¼ cup | 17 | 1 |
| Quinces | 1 avg. | 40 | 3 |
| Raisins (seedless) | 1 TB | 60 | 3 |
| Raspberries | ¼ cup | 21 | 0 |
| Tangerines | 1 avg. | 35 | 16 |
| Watermelon | 1 thick slice | 13 | 0 |
| | | | |
| *Grains and Related Products* | | | |
| Barley | ¼ cup | 200 | 15 |
| Cereals (no sugar or salt added) | | | |
|   Cornflakes | ½ cup | 84 | 1 |
|   Cornmeal (c) | ½ cup | 30 | 0 |
|   Cream of wheat (c) | ½ cup | 60 | 0 |
|   Farina (c) | ½ cup | 68 | 0 |
|   Granola (no coconut or | | | |
|     coconut/palm oils) | 3 TB | 110 | 0 |
|   Maltex (c) | ½ cup | 71 | 3 |
|   Millet grits (c) | ½ cup | 60 | 2 |
|   Millet, puffed | ½ cup | 60 | 2 |
|   Oats, rolled (c) | ½ cup | 77 | 0 |
|   Ralston (c) | ½ cup | 77 | 0 |
|   Rice, puffed | ½ cup | 39 | 0 |
|   Wheat, puffed | ½ cup | 27 | 1 |

| Food | Unit or Measure | Calories | Sodium† |
|------|-----------------|----------|---------|
| Wheat, shredded | 1 biscuit | 50 | 4 |
| Wheatena (c) | ½ cup | 103 | 0 |
| Wheat germ | 1 TB | 28 | 1 |
| Kasha (buckwheat groats) | ¼ cup | 86 | 0 |
| Rice | | | |
|   Brown | ¼ cup | 212 | 1 |
|   Instant | ¼ cup | 214 | 0 |
|   White (enriched) | ½ cup | 213 | 0 |

*Herbs, Spices, and Extracts*
In the amounts used, calories are 0 and sodium is 0. Do not use garlic salt, celery salt, or celery flakes; they are high in sodium. Opt for chili con carne *seasoning* (per teaspoon—calories 0, sodium 1) instead of chili con carne *powder* (calories 0, sodium 57). Avoid extracts to which sugar has been added.

*Jams and Jellies*

| | | | |
|------|-----------------|----------|---------|
| Commercial (sweetened with honey only) | 1 TB | 55 | 1 |

*Meat*
Beef

| | | | |
|------|-----------------|----------|---------|
|   Chuck | 4 oz. | 181 | 74 |
|   Double bone sirloin | 4 oz. | 181 | 74 |
|   Filet mignon | 4 oz. | 187 | 74 |
|   Flank steak | 4 oz. | 163 | 74 |
|   London broil (hindshank) | 4 oz. | 154 | 74 |
|   Porterhouse | 4 oz. | 187 | 74 |
|   Pot roast (foreshank) | 4 oz. | 161 | 74 |
|   Roast beef (round) | 4 oz. | 155 | 74 |
|   Rump | 4 oz. | 181 | 74 |
|   Shell steak | 4 oz. | 187 | 74 |
|   Short plate | 4 oz. | 187 | 74 |
|   Sirloin | 4 oz. | 163 | 74 |
|   Tailsteak | 4 oz. | 187 | 74 |
|   T-bone | 4 oz. | 163 | 74 |
| Ham (fresh boneless) | 4 oz. | 144 | 80 |
| Lamb | | | |
|   Leg | 4 oz. | 148 | 70 |
|   Loin chops and other loin cuts | 4 oz. | 157 | 70 |
|   Rib chops | 4 oz. | 181 | 70 |
|   Shoulder chops | 4 oz. | 169 | 70 |
| Pork (picnic) | 4 oz. | 155 | 70 |
| Rabbit | 4 oz. | 140 | 53 |
| Veal | | | |
|   Leg | 4 oz. | 149 | 90 |
|   Loin chops and other loin cuts | 4 oz. | 178 | 90 |

| Food | Unit or Measure | Calories | Sodium† | |
|---|---|---|---|---|
| Veal | | | | |
|   Round and rump | 4 oz. | 160 | 90 | |
|   Shoulder chops and chuck | 4 oz. | 160 | 90 | |
| Venison | 4 oz. | 112 | 90 | (E) |
| | | | | |
| *Oils, Fats, and Salad Dressings* | | | | |
| Almond oil | 1 TB | 120 | 0 | |
| All-purpose oil | 1 TB | 120 | 0 | |
| Apricot kernel oil | 1 TB | 120 | 0 | |
| Corn oil | 1 TB | 120 | 0 | |
| Cottonseed oil | 1 TB | 120 | 0 | |
| Margarine (tub, liquid corn oil, no salt added) | 1 TB | 102 | | |
| Mayonnaise (commercial eggless, low-sodium) | 1 TB | 92 | 6 | |
| Olive oil | 1 TB | 120 | 0 | |
| Safflower oil | 1 TB | 120 | 0 | |
| Salad dressing (haute cuisine of health) | 1 TB | 62 | 1 | |
| Soybean oil | 1 TB | 120 | 0 | |
| Sunflower oil | 1 TB | 120 | 0 | |
| Walnut oil | 1 TB | 120 | 0 | |
| | | | | |
| *Pasta* | | | | |
| Macaroni (no salt added) | 2 oz. | 210 | 1 | |
| Spaghetti (no salt added) | 2 oz. | 210 | 2 | |
| | | | | |
| *Poultry* | | | | |
| Chicken (fryers without skin) | | | | |
|   Light meat (other than breast) | 4 oz. | 115 | 62 | |
|   Light meat (breast) | 4 oz. | 126 | 89 | |
|   Dark meat (other than leg) | 4 oz. | 128 | 91 | |
|   Dark meat (leg) | 4 oz. | 146 | 125 | |
| Turkey | | | | |
|   Mature (dark meat) | 4 oz. | 145 | 81 | |
|   Mature (white meat) | 4 oz. | 130 | 51 | |
|   Young (dark meat) | 4 oz. | 127 | 81 | |
|   Young (white meat) | 4 oz. | 123 | 51 | |
| | | | | |
| *Sweeteners* | | | | |
| Carob, powder | ¼ cup | 110 | 3 | |
| Honey | 1 TB | 62 | 2 | |
| | | | | |
| *Thickeners* | | | | |
| Arrowroot | 1 TB | 30 | 1 | (E) |
| Cornstarch | 1 TB | 29 | 1 | |

| Food | Unit or Measure | Calories | Sodium† | |
|------|-----------------|----------|---------|---|
| *Vegetables* | | | | |
| Artichokes | | | | |
|   French | 1 med. | 48 | 42 | (E) |
|   French, hearts | 1 med. | 7 | 13 | |
|   Jerusalem | 1 med. | 4 | 15 | (E) |
| Asparagus | | | | |
|   Stalks | 1 med. | 2 | 0 | |
|   Spears (cut into ½" pieces) | ¼ cup | 18 | 2 | |
|   Spears (as above, frozen) | ¼ cup | 18 | 2 | |
| Bamboo shoots | 4 oz. | 35 | 10 | (E) |
| Beans | | | | |
|   Green | ¼ cup | 12 | 1 | |
|   Kidney | ¼ cup | 200 | 1 | |
|   Lima | ¼ cup | 50 | 5 | |
|   Navy | ¼ cup | 174 | 8 | |
|   Wax (yellow) | ¼ cup | 12 | 5 | |
|   White (marrow) | ¼ cup | 160 | 2 | |
| Bean curd | 4 oz. | 158 | 4 | |
| Bean sprouts | | | | |
|   Mung | ¼ cup | 8 | 1 | |
|   Soy | ¼ cup | 18 | 1 | |
| Beets (diced) | ¼ cup | 14 | 18 | |
| Broccoli (chopped) | ¼ cup | 11 | 5 | |
| Brussels sprouts | ¼ cup | 22 | 12 | |
| Cabbage (shredded) | ¼ cup | 5 | 3 | |
|   Chinese (shredded) | ¼ cup | 6 | 3 | |
| Carrots (grated or shredded) | ¼ cup | 12 | 13 | |
| Cauliflower | ¼ cup | 8 | 9 | |
| Celery (diced) | ¼ cup | 5 | 38 | |
| Chives | 1 TB | 1 | 0 | |
| Chick-peas (garbanzos) | ¼ cup | 188 | 13 | |
| Chicory | 1 leaf | 3 | 1 | |
| Corn | ¼ cup | 38 | 0 | |
| Cucumbers | ¼ cup | 4 | 2 | |
| Eggplant | ¼ cup | 7 | 1 | |
| Endive | 1 leaf | 2 | 1 | |
| Escarole | 1 leaf | 1 | 1 | |
| Garlic | 1 clove | 6 | 1 | |
| Horseradish (unprepared) | 1 oz. | 87 | 8 | |
| Leeks | ¼ cup | 5 | 1 | |
| Lentils | ¼ cup | 62 | 1 | |
| Lettuce | 1 leaf | 1 | 1 | |
| Mushrooms | 1 large | 3 | 15 | |
| Mustard greens | ¼ cup | 8 | 2 | |
| Okra | ¼ cup | 9 | 1 | |

| Food | Unit or Measure | Calories | Sodium† |
|---|---|---|---|
| Onion (grated or minced) | ¼ cup | 20 | 6 |
| Peas | | | |
|   Shelled | ¼ cup | 28 | 5 |
|   Split (dried) | ¼ cup | 172 | 13 |
| Peppers (green or red) | ¼ cup | 6 | 3 |
| Popcorn | | | |
|   Popped (no salt or butter added) | ¼ cup | 6 | 0 |
|   Unpopped | 1 TB | 76 | 1 |
| Potatoes | | | |
|   Sweet | 1 avg. | 183 | 12 |
|   White | 1 avg. | 110 | 11 |
| Radishes | 1 avg. | 3 | 2 |
| Rhubarb (diced) | ¼ cup | 20 | 2 |
| Shallots | 1 avg. | 9 | 2 |
| Spinach | ¼ cup | 23 | 83 |
| Squash | | | |
|   Summer | ¼ cup | 23 | 0 |
|   Winter | ¼ cup | 15 | 0 |
| Tofu (bean curd) | 4 oz. | 158 | 8 |
| Tomatoes | | | |
|   Canned (no salt added) | ¼ cup | 13 | 8 |
|   Fresh | 1 avg. | 30 | 3 |
| Tomato paste (no salt added) * | 1 TB | 18 | 9 |
| Tomato purée (no salt added) | 1 TB | 1 | 2 |
| Turnip greens (c) | ¼ cup | 11 | 3 |
| Turnips (yellow) (c) | ¼ cup | 13 | 3 |
| Yams | 1 avg. | 200 | 15 (E) |
| Zucchini | ¼ cup | 4 | 1 |

* Foods listed are raw, except where otherwise noted by symbol (c).
† Sodium is measured in milligrams.
‡ E = Estimated.

# 2

# HAUTE CUISINE
# OF HEALTH RECIPES

Cooking is a great creative experience. That's true even if you've never cooked before. Start by following one of my recipes to get the feel of it, to learn the joy of creating a superlative dish from healthful ingredients. Then, next time, adjust the recipe to your likes and dislikes—only you know the flavors you prefer—and make every morsel taste the way you dreamed it should taste. Call what you're doing a search—a search for the perfect dish. You can find it.

And, oh, the rewards! That feeling of creative joy! You think that only artists and writers can feel it? You can, too. You need no special training, no inspiration, no talent. All you need is your own kitchen and a desire to feel a sense of accomplishment. My simple, but elegant, recipes will lead you into new bright hours of self-fulfillment.

There are so many other rewards. There's the feeling of stardom that comes from the applause of your family and friends. "That's *so* delicious! How did you *ever* do it!" is like getting an Oscar. There's the feeling of relaxation that so many of us search for everywhere in this busy-busy world; and you find it right in your own kitchen. There are few activities that shut out the clamor of the world as totally and pleasantly as cooking. Cooking *work*? Not when it's done

*my* way. Then it's a refreshment of the body and the spirit.

And what about the rewards to your palate? When my husband and I travel here and abroad promoting our books, lecturing, and demonstrating, we taste the foods of world-famous chefs. But after a while the food cloys. There's a sameness, a monotony, a poverty of ideas. It seems to us that even *les specialités de la maison* are cooked to formula. But when healthful ingredients are cooked my way, there's a virtually unending flow of novel flavors—flavors you never before thought existed.

Economic rewards? Why, certainly. Why pay the skyrocketing costs of restaurants when you can eat inexpensively at home—and eat better?

But the best reward is still to come. My cuisine nourishes you, slims you, vitalizes you. It helps free you from the fears of diseases related to faulty nutrition. It gives you a sense of control over your health; you are not letting things happen to your body and mind, you are making them happen—wonderful things. My cuisine makes you feel *good*. The joys of cooking my way can bring you the reward that men and women have sought for thousands of years—a sound mind in a sound body.

And learning to cook my way is a reward in itself—it's such *fun*. Cook for yourself. Cook for your family (they'll soon forget there's any other way *to* cook). And teach your youngsters to cook this way. The future belongs to them. Let them approach it lean, vigorous, and clear minded. It's the best heritage you can give them. Your fun time in the kitchen could mean great times for you and everyone you hold dear.

# HOW TO USE THESE RECIPES

When the reducing, binge-ing, or maintenance menu calls for a chicken dish, use a chicken recipe; for a meat dish, a meat recipe; for a dessert, a dessert recipe; and so on. It's *that* simple.

You don't have to count calories; it's been done for you. You don't have to worry about sodium, cholesterol, or any other nutrient; the right amounts have been incorporated into each dish. Plan your three major meals with these recipes, and your daily nutrient intake will conform closely to standards set by government nutrition authorities.

Good cooking and good health!

# MEAT

## STEAK WITH BROWN SAUCE

Sauté a lean and tender sirloin, baby it with a generous showering of herbs and spices, and sit down to a steak that for tastiness, beefiness and texture rivals that to be found in the world's greatest restaurants.

1½ pounds lean boneless sirloin, cut 1 inch thick

½ teaspoon each dried thyme and rosemary leaves, crushed, and ground ginger

2 teaspoons each corn oil and Italian olive oil, combined

2 large cloves garlic, minced

2 large shallots, minced

1 tablespoon minced sweet green pepper

4 large fresh mushrooms, washed, dried, trimmed, and coarsely chopped

⅓ cup Miracle Chicken Stock (page 168)

3 tablespoons dry vermouth

2 teaspoons tomato paste (no salt added)

1. Wipe meat with paper toweling. Sprinkle and rub with herbs and ginger.

2. Heat 2 teaspoons combined oils in well-seasoned iron skillet (see note below) until hot. Sauté steak for 5 minutes over medium heat on each side. Turn twice more and sauté for 1 to 2 minutes on each side. (Do not overcook; steak will be medium rare). Transfer to warmed serving plate. Cover with waxed paper.

3. To prepare sauce, heat balance of oil in skillet. Sauté garlic, shallots, green pepper, and mushrooms until lightly browned, stirring constantly so that mixture does not stick to skillet.

4. Combine stock, vermouth, and tomato paste. Add to skillet. Scrape skillet to loosen browned particles. Stir and cook sauce over medium-high heat until reduced by half. Finished sauce will be thick.

5. Pour exuded juices from steak into skillet. Stir to blend. Pour over steak and serve immediately, slicing steak at table.

YIELD: Serves 4

NOTE: For directions on how to prepare a well-seasoned iron skillet, see note for Savory Sautéed Chicken on page 130.

## BEST-EVER SKILLET BEEFBURGERS

Sprinkle with chili, add just the right amount of herbs and spices, and prepare yourself for the most exciting-flavored hamburger you've ever tasted. Sheer luxury! And child's play to make.

1 pound ground extra-lean beef
⅓ cup soft bread crumbs (preferably salt-free)
1 teaspoon each chili con carne seasoning (no salt or pepper added) and ground coriander
8 dashes ground red (cayenne) pepper
1 teaspoon dried basil leaves, crushed
1 tablespoon minced fresh parsley
3 teaspoons corn oil
3 large shallots, minced
2 large cloves garlic, minced
¼ cup dry red wine

1. Combine beef, crumbs, spices, and herbs in bowl. Blend well.

2. Heat 1 teaspoon oil in nonstick skillet until hot. Add 1 minced shallot and all of garlic. Sauté just until wilted.

Add wine. Cook for 30 seconds. Pour into meat mixture. Blend. Shape into 4 patties.

3. Heat balance of oil in skillet. Spread balance of minced shallots over skillet. Lay patties on top, flattening with spatula to ½-inch thickness. Sauté until browned on both sides. (Do not overcook; meat should be crisp on the outside and lightly pink on the inside.) Serve immediately.

YIELD: Serves 4

VARIATION: Substitute ¼ cup Miracle Chicken Stock (page 168) for wine and add 1 teaspoon tomato paste (no salt added) in step 2.

## SAUTEED VEAL PATTIES

Ground veal by itself is fairly bland. Here it happily accepts the flavors of meaty mushrooms, sweet carrot, and tart apple—and comes to your table brimming with exceptional flavor and texture.

4 teaspoons corn oil
2 large shallots, minced
2 large cloves garlic, minced
3 large fresh mushrooms, washed, dried, trimmed, and coarsely chopped
½ tart green apple, peeled and coarsely chopped
1 tablespoon grated carrot
¼ cup red wine
6 dashes ground red (cayenne) pepper
½ teaspoon chili con carne seasoning (no salt or pepper added)
½ teaspoon dried thyme leaves, crushed
1 pound ground lean veal
1½ tablespoons toasted wheat germ (no sugar added)
2 tablespoons lightly toasted bread crumbs (see note, page 121)

1. Heat 2 teaspoons oil in nonstick skillet until hot. Add shallots, garlic, and mushrooms and sauté for 2 minutes, stirring constantly. Add apple and carrot. Sauté for 1 minute. Add wine, spices, and thyme, stirring to blend. Set aside.

2. Combine veal with wheat germ and bread crumbs in bowl. Add sautéed ingredients and blend. Shape into 8 patties ½ inch thick. Wipe out skillet.

3. Heat balance of oil (2 teaspoons) in skillet until hot. Add patties and sauté over medium-high heat until golden brown on both sides. (Do not overcook; meat should be crisp on the outside and lightly pink inside.) Serve immediately.

YIELD: Serves 4

## LUSCIOUS LEG OF LAMB

This recipe and the next introduce you to new and exotic ways to prepare leg of lamb— the lowest in fat of all lamb cuts. Leg of lamb, bone in, is roasted to a dark, rosy-hued lusciousness with chili, herbs, and tomato paste. The roasted filleted leg, subtly sweetened with fruit and mint, seems not like lamb at all, but some new creation to pamper your palate.

3 large cloves garlic, minced
½ teaspoon each dried rosemary, thyme, and sage leaves, crushed
½ teaspoon dry mustard
2 teaspoons chili con carne seasoning (no salt or pepper added)
8 dashes ground red (cayenne) pepper
2 tablespoons each apple juice (no sugar added), corn oil, and wine vinegar
2 teaspoons tomato paste (no salt added)
½ leg of lamb, preferably shank end (3½ pounds) well trimmed
½ cup Miracle Chicken Stock (page 168)
Minced fresh parsley

1. Prepare marinade by combining first 7 listed ingredients in small bowl. Blend. (Mixture will be thick).

2. Wipe meat with damp paper toweling, then again with dry paper toweling. Tear off large sheet of heavy-duty aluminum foil. Lay lamb on top. Spread with marinade, turning to coat. Close foil tightly. Place in refrigerator and let marinate for 6 hours or more. Bring to room temperature before roasting.

3. Place meat on rack in shallow roasting pan. Roast, uncovered, in preheated 400°F oven for 15 minutes. Baste with one third of stock. Reduce heat to 350°F. Roast for 40 to 50 minutes, basting twice more with balance of stock at 20-minute intervals (see note below). (Do not overcook; meat will be medium rare.)

4. Slice thin and serve, spooned with pan juices and sprinkled with parsley.

YIELD: Serves 6

NOTE: Roasting time may vary slightly with thickness of meat and bone.

## ROAST FILLET OF LAMB

2 pounds fillet of lamb, in one piece, well trimmed, rolled 4 inches in diameter (see note)
¼ cup each orange and pineapple juice (no sugar added)
1 tablespoon apple cider vinegar
2 large cloves garlic, minced
2 large shallots, minced
1 teaspoon peeled and minced fresh ginger
1 tablespoon minced fresh mint, tarragon, or rosemary leaves
6 dashes ground red (cayenne) pepper
Peeled navel orange slices for garnish

1. Wipe meat with paper toweling. Prick in several places with thin skewer. Place in bowl.
2. Combine balance of ingredients, except garnish, in jar. Shake well to blend. Pour over meat, turning to coat. Let marinate for at least 1 hour. (Meat may be tightly covered and refrigerated overnight. Remove from refrigerator 1 hour before roasting.) Drain meat. Pour marinade into saucepan.

3. Place meat on rack in shallow roasting pan. Roast, uncovered, in preheated 400°F oven for 45 minutes. Remove from oven. Cover with waxed paper and let stand for 5 minutes before slicing.
4. Bring marinade to simmering point. Simmer for 5 minutes, uncovered. Strain into sauceboat. Slice meat thin and serve, garnished with orange slices, along with strained hot marinade.

YIELD: Serves 4

VARIATION: Pour strained marinade back into saucepan. Add ⅓ cup dry red wine. Simmer for 7 minutes. Pour into sauceboat and serve.

NOTE: Many supermarkets feature boned and rolled leg of lamb. It slices best when made from the shank end (the leanest, meatiest, and juiciest part). If the shank end is not on display, ask for it.

## HERBED ROAST PORK

Here's an example of a new, simple, and delicious approach to roasting meats. Try it, and watch an otherwise plain roast turn into an ecstatically delicious, fork-tender delight.

2 pounds lean boned and rolled pork (4 inches in diameter)
1 recipe Herb Marinade I (page 164)
Minced fresh parsley

1. Wipe meat with paper toweling. Place in large bowl. Pour marinade over meat, turning well to coat. Let stand for at least 1 hour at room temperature (or overnight, tightly covered and refrigerated), turning often. Drain meat, reserving marinade.

2. Place meat on rack in shallow roasting pan. Cover loosely with aluminum foil. Roast in preheated 375°F oven for 30 minutes. Uncover. Spoon with one third of marinade. Re-cover and roast for 30 minutes. Repeat basting and roasting procedure twice more at 20-minute intervals until done (total cooking time is 1½ to 1¾ hours; pork must be cooked well done).

3. Remove from oven. Cover and let stand for 10 minutes before slicing. Slice thin and serve sprinkled with minced fresh parsley.

YIELD: Serves 4

NOTES:

1. The diameter of a roast, not its weight, governs cooking time. For example, a 4-inch-diameter roast takes the same time to cook whether it weighs 4 pounds or 6 pounds.

2. Roasting time for lamb, veal, or beef, varies with degree of doneness. Oven time for any of these meats, done medium-rare (my preference), is 1¼ to 1½ hours. For timing your roast accurately, use a meat thermometer.

3. If roast is refrigerated for any length of time, let stand at room temperature for 1 hour before placing in oven.

## ROSEMARY VEAL CHOPS

Rosemary, a hearty, fragrant relative of mint, adds special luster to chicken, veal, and marinades. The fresh variety is best, but dried rosemary is excellent when crushed well in a mortar and pestle. If you've never used rosemary before, be prepared for an exquisite and distinctive new flavor. You'll love it in this veal dish.

½ ounce dried imported dark mushrooms
¼ cup water
4 loin or rib veal chops (1½ pounds), well trimmed
2 teaspoons dried rosemary leaves, crushed
8 dashes ground red (cayenne) pepper
2 teaspoons each corn oil and Italian olive oil, combined
3 large cloves garlic, minced
1 medium onion, minced
1 small sweet red pepper, seeded and cut into ¼-inch slivers
¼ cup each apple juice (no sugar added) and dry vermouth, combined
1 tart apple, peeled, cored, and thickly sliced
1 tablespoon minced fresh parsley

1. Break mushrooms into small pieces. Soak in ¼ cup water until soft (about 30 minutes).

2. Wipe meat with paper toweling. Rub with rosemary and ground red pepper. Heat half of combined oils in well-seasoned iron skillet (see note below) until hot. Brown meat lightly on both sides. (Watch heat under skillet carefully and lower if meat begins to stick; do not add more oil.) Transfer to plate.

3. Heat balance of oil (2 teaspoons) in skillet. Add garlic, onion, and sweet red pepper. Sauté until lightly browned. Add apple juice—vermouth mixture, scraping skillet to loosen browned particles. Add mushrooms and soaking liquid. Return meat to skillet, arranging in one layer. Spoon with juices and vegetables. Cover tightly and simmer for 20 minutes.

4. Add apple. Re-cover and simmer for 20 minutes. Remove from heat. Let stand, covered, for 10 minutes. Serve on individual warmed plates, sprinkled with minced fresh parsley and spooned with sauce and apples.

YIELD: Serves 4

VARIATION: Lean, boned stewing veal (1½ pounds) may be substituted for chops. Add 3 tablespoons Miracle Chicken Stock (page 168) to recipe and reduce apple juice to 2 tablespoons.

NOTE: For directions on how to prepare a well-seasoned iron skillet, see note for Savory Sautéed Chicken on page 130.

## ORANGE VEAL SCALLOPINI

Try my adventurous herbed and fruit-sauced version of a classical Italian favorite. It will open up a whole new glorious and exciting world of flavors to you.

4 slices veal (1½ pounds), cut from the leg, pounded to ¼-inch thickness
2 tablespoons fresh lemon juice
1 teaspoon dried rosemary leaves, crushed
½ teaspoon ground ginger
1½ teaspoons each corn oil and Italian olive oil, combined
2 large cloves garlic, minced
3 large shallots, minced
1 tablespoon minced sweet green pepper
2 tablespoons each dry vermouth, Miracle Chicken Stock (page 168), and partially thawed orange juice concentrate (no sugar added)
½ teaspoon dry mustard
2 tablespoons evaporated skim milk

1. Wipe veal with paper toweling. Place in bowl. Sprinkle with lemon juice, turning to coat. Let stand for 30 minutes. Pat again with paper toweling. Sprinkle and rub with rosemary and ginger.

2. Heat combined oils in well-seasoned iron skillet (see note below) until hot. Add garlic, shallots, and green pepper, spreading evenly across skillet. Sauté for 30 seconds. Lay meat on top of minced ingredients. Sauté over medium-high heat until lightly browned on both sides (about 2 minutes on each side).

3. Combine vermouth, stock, orange juice concentrate, and mustard in cup. Blend well. Pour over veal. Turn meat several times to coat evenly. Bring to simmering point. Transfer meat to warmed serving plate. Cover to keep warm.

4. Turn up heat under skillet and reduce sauce by one third. Turn off heat. Stir in evaporated milk. Spoon over veal and serve immediately.

YIELD: Serves 4

VARIATION: For a more orange-y flavor, in step 3 add ½ teaspoon grated orange rind (preferably from navel orange).

NOTE: For directions on how to prepare a well-seasoned iron skillet, see note for Savory Sautéed Chicken on page 130.

## STIR-FRIED STEAK AND BROCCOLI

Enjoy a new, exciting experience—cooking with a wok. Here's how to do it:

Season your wok according to manufacturer's directions. Read recipe several times before cooking. Prepare ingredients and place them in containers near stove in the order in which they will be used. You'll have no time to hunt and peck after you've started cooking. Hint: Gather your family around the table *before* you start to cook. This food can't wait. (For more detailed instructions for getting the most from your wok, and for more delicious slimming recipes, see *Francine Prince's New Gourmet Recipes for Dieters.*)

1½ cups fresh broccoli flowerets
1 egg white
2 teaspoons cornstarch
8 dashes ground red (cayenne) pepper
2 teaspoons dry vermouth
1½ pounds lean, tender boneless sirloin or flank steak, cut into 2½-inch by ½-inch strips
1 teaspoon each medium-dry sherry and water
2 teaspoons tomato paste (no salt added)
½ teaspoon each dried thyme and tarragon leaves, crushed
2 teaspoons each corn oil and Italian olive oil, combined
2 large cloves garlic, minced
1½ teaspoons peeled and shredded fresh ginger
4 large fresh mushrooms, washed, dried, trimmed, and thinly sliced
½ cup Miracle Chicken Stock (page 168)
2 teaspoons water

1. Parboil broccoli flowerets by dropping into a pot of rapidly boiling water and cooking for 1 minute. Drain in colander. Place colander under cold running water to stop cooking action. Set aside.

2. Combine egg white, 1 teaspoon cornstarch, ground red pepper, and vermouth in bowl. Beat with fork to blend. Add meat. Turn until well coated. Cover and let stand for 10 minutes.

3. Combine sherry, water, tomato paste, and dried herbs in small bowl. Stir to blend. Set aside.

4. Heat wok over high heat for 1½ minutes. Pour half of combined oils around rim of wok. Add half each of garlic and ginger. Stir-fry for 30 seconds. Add meat. Stir-fry for 2 minutes. Transfer contents of wok to open plate.

5. Add balance of oil (2 teaspoons) to rim of wok. Add balance of garlic and ginger. Stir-fry for 30 seconds. Add broccoli and mushrooms. Stir-fry for 1 minute.

6. Return meat mixture to wok. Add stock. Cover and cook over medium heat for 1 minute. Remove cover.

7. Dissolve balance of cornstarch (1 teaspoon) in 2 teaspoons water. Add to mixture, stirring until slightly thickened.

8. Turn onto serving plate. Serve immediately.

YIELD: Serves 4

# FISH

### DELICIOUS BAKED CRISP FILLET OF LEMON SOLE

Sole is everyone's favorite even when it's simply broiled, as it usually is, with butter and salt. Imagine then, how much you'll love my version, flavor enhanced with a zesty marinade and crisped to perfection with my tasty crumb mixture. Plain old broiled fillet of sole will become just a memory.

1½ pounds fresh lemon sole fillets, cut into serving pieces
2 tablespoons fresh lime juice
3 teaspoons partially thawed orange juice concentrate (no sugar added)
¼ teaspoon grated orange rind, preferably from navel orange
1 tablespoon dry vermouth
1 large shallot, minced
¼ cup lightly toasted bread crumbs (see note below)
2 tablespoons toasted wheat germ (no sugar added)
⅛ teaspoon ground cinnamon
6 dashes ground red (cayenne) pepper
3 dashes ground cloves
½ teaspoon corn oil for pan, plus 2 teaspoons

1. Wash fish and pat dry with paper toweling. Place in shallow bowl.

2. Prepare marinade by combining lime juice, 1 teaspoon orange juice concentrate, grated orange rind, vermouth, and shallot in jar, shaking to blend. Pour over fish, turning fish to coat. Let stand for 15 to 30 minutes at room temperature, turning twice.

3. Combine bread crumbs, wheat germ, cinnamon, ground red pepper, and cloves in wide bowl, stirring to blend. Drain fillets, pouring marinade into saucepan. Dip fillets into crumb mixture, coating well, then shaking off excess.

4. Lightly oil shallow baking pan large enough to accommodate fish in one layer. Place pan in preheated 400°F oven for 5 minutes. Remove from oven. Place fillets in hot pan in one layer. Bake for 5 to 6 minutes. Turn. Bake for an additional 5 to 6 minutes. Fish should be crisply browned on the outside and moist on the inside. Baking time will vary with thickness of fillets.

5. While fish is baking on second side, prepare easy sauce. Add balance of orange juice concentrate (2 teaspoons) and 2 teaspoons oil to saucepan with marinade. Bring to simmering point. Simmer over very low heat for 3 minutes. Strain. Serve in sauceboat along with baked fish.

YIELD: Serves 4

NOTE: To prepare about ½ cup bread crumbs, cut 4 slices of unsalted bread into small cubes. Toast lightly. Place in electric blender or food processor. Process until fine. (For additional salt-free bread recipes, see *The Dieter's Gourmet Cookbook* and *Francine Prince's New Gourmet Recipes for Dieters.*)

## DELICATE HALIBUT FILLETS

If you've never liked fish any way but deep fried, try my version of filleted halibut. Marinated in vinegar and spices, coated with crumbs and herbs, and then sautéed to a butternut brown, it reaches new and exciting culinary heights both in flavor and texture. You'll never miss fried fish again!

1½ pounds halibut fillets (cut from small fish)
2 tablespoons each apple juice (no sugar added), wine vinegar, and dry vermouth
1 tablespoon minced fresh dill
2 cloves garlic, minced
1 large shallot, minced
½ teaspoon ground ginger
8 dashes ground red (cayenne) pepper
1½ teaspoons dried rosemary leaves, crushed
½ cup unseasoned bread crumbs (preferably no salt added)
2 teaspoons each corn oil and Italian olive oil, combined
Lemon wedges for garnish

1. Wash fish and pat dry with paper toweling. Combine next 6 listed ingredients in bowl, stirring to blend. Add fish, turning to coat. Let marinate at room temperature for 30 minutes, turning twice.

2. Remove fish from marinade. Drain on paper toweling. Pour marinade into strainer. Spoon solids in strainer onto fillets, distributing evenly and pressing into fish. Set aside.

3. Combine and stir crushed rosemary with crumbs. Sprinkle half of mixture onto large flat plate. Lay fillets on top of crumbs, pressing into mixture. Pour balance of crumbs over fillets, coating well. If time permits, refrigerate for 30 minutes before cooking. This will encourage crumbs to adhere to fish.

4. Heat half of combined oils in large nonstick skillet until hot. Sauté fillets on one side over medium heat for 3 minutes, or until lightly browned. Add balance of oils (2 teaspoons), turn, and sauté until butternut brown. (Do not overcook.) Serve immediately on warmed individual plates garnished with lemon wedges.

YIELD: Serves 4

VARIATION: The ingredients in this recipe marry particularly well with halibut, but you can successfully substitute fillet of lemon sole or flounder.

## SUBLIME FILLET OF SEA BASS

Sea bass (preferably the white variety) is a sweet, firmly textured fish, with which most Americans are not familiar. Here's a delicious and quick way for you to get acquainted with this nonpareil gift from the sea.

¼ cup dry vermouth
1 teaspoon each fresh lemon juice and wine vinegar
4 teaspoons minced fresh dill
1½ pounds fresh white sea bass fillets, cut into 4 serving pieces
½ teaspoon sweet (unsalted) 100 percent corn oil margarine for pan
2 large shallots, minced
1 large clove garlic, minced
8 dashes ground red (cayenne) pepper
6 teaspoons lightly toasted bread crumbs (see Note page 121)
2 teaspoons each melted margarine and corn oil, combined
Lime wedges for garnish

1. Prepare easy marinade by combining vermouth, lemon juice, vinegar, and 2 teaspoons dill in bowl, stirring to blend.

2. Wash fish under cold running water and pat dry with paper toweling. Add to marinade, turning several times to coat. Let stand at room temperature for 15 minutes, turning twice. Drain, reserving marinade.

3. Place fillets in lightly margarine-greased pan large enough to accommodate fish in one layer. Sprinkle with shallots and garlic, then spoon with 2 tablespoons marinade. Sprinkle with ground red pepper and bread crumbs. Drizzle with combined corn oil and melted margarine.

4. Bake in preheated 400°F oven for 6 minutes. Then place fish under broiler and broil for 5 minutes. (Fish should flake easily when tested with fork; cooking time will vary with thickness of fillets.) Serve on individual warmed plates, sprinkled with balance of dill and garnished with lime wedges.

YIELD: Serves 4

NOTE: Fresh herbs taste best in this recipe. If fresh dill is not available, substitute fresh tarragon or basil.

## SHRIMP-STUFFED STRIPED BASS

Here is an exquisite combination of both finny and finless sea food, flavored with vermouth's garden of herbs and accented with minty rosemary. One woman said to me, "This isn't dieting. This is heaven."

2 striped bass (1½ pounds each), cleaned, heads left on
½ pound fresh shrimp, shelled and deveined, coarsely chopped
2 tablespoons fresh lime juice
1 teaspoon tarragon vinegar
3 teaspoons corn oil, plus ½ teaspoon for pan
2 cloves garlic, minced
3 large shallots, minced
2 tablespoons dry vermouth, plus ¼ cup
2 tablespoons grated carrot
½ cup soft bread crumbs (preferably salt-free)
1½ teaspoons dried rosemary leaves, crushed
½ teaspoon ground marjoram
2 tablespoons minced fresh parsley
8 dashes red (cayenne) pepper
1 large onion, thinly sliced
Lemon wedges and parsley sprigs for garnish

1. Rinse fish inside and out under cold running water. Dry with paper toweling. Wash and dry cleaned shrimps. Make 3 gashes across each fish on both sides. Lay fish and shrimp in rectangular baking pan.

2. Combine lime juice and vinegar. Pour over fish and shrimp, turning to coat, and rubbing liquid into cavity and gashes. Let stand for 30 minutes to 1 hour.

3. Heat 2 teaspoons oil in nonstick skillet until hot. Sauté garlic and shallots for 2 minutes, taking care not to brown. Add the 2 tablespoons vermouth. Cook for 30 seconds. Turn into bowl.

4. Drain shrimp and add to bowl; add carrot, bread crumbs, 1 teaspoon rosemary, the marjoram, 1 tablespoon parsley, and 4 dashes ground red pepper. Stir to combine ingredients.

5. Drain fish. Blot inside and out with paper toweling. Fill cavity with shrimp mixture. Secure with skewers. Brush fish with balance of oil (1 teaspoon). Sprinkle and rub with balance of rosemary (½ teaspoon) and ground red pepper (4 dashes).

6. Wipe out baking pan. Line with heavy-duty aluminum foil. Brush foil lightly with ½ teaspoon oil. Lay fish in baking pan. Cover each fish with sliced onion. Sprinkle with balance of parsley (1 tablespoon). Cover tightly with another sheet of aluminum foil and bake in preheated 400°F oven for 12 minutes. Remove foil. Pour the ¼ cup vermouth over fish. Baste with pan juices several times. Re-cover with foil and bake for 8 to 9 minutes, or until fish flakes easily when tested with fork.

7. Lay fish on warmed serving platter. Pour cooking liquid over fish. Garnish with lemon wedges and parsley sprigs and serve individual portions of fish and stuffing at table.

YIELD: Serves 4

## SUPER-DELICIOUS BROILED TILEFISH

Tilefish, a recently popularized denizen of the deep, is one of the lowest in fat of all fish (a mere 7 percent in terms of total calories). Its skin resembles old-time colorful linoleum. Because it feeds on crustacea, it has some of the flavor and texture of lobster. It excels here enrobed in a sauce of tart and sweet fruit juices, chili, and herbs.

2 tablespoons each fresh lime juice, orange juice, and dry vermouth
8 dashes ground red (cayenne) pepper
2 tilefish steaks (1½ pounds), each slice cut in half along length of bone
½ teaspoon dried sage leaves, crushed
1 teaspoon chili con carne seasoning (no salt or pepper added)
2 teaspoons corn oil
1 large leek, white part only, well washed, dried, and minced
1 medium onion, minced
1 tablespoon minced fresh parsley

1. Combine lime juice, orange juice, vermouth, and ground red pepper in bowl.

2. Wash fish and dry thoroughly with paper toweling. Place in bowl with liquid mixture, turning well to coat. Let marinate at room temperature for 30 minutes, turning often. Drain, reserving marinade. Pat with paper toweling. Sprinkle and rub fish on both sides with sage and chili con carne seasoning.

3. Heat oil in nonstick skillet until hot. Sauté leek and onion until just wilted (do not brown). Spread half of mixture across shallow broiling pan. Lay fish on top. Spoon fish with balance of sautéed mixture, then spoon each slice of fish with a tablespoon of marinade.

4. Broil 6 inches from heat for 7 minutes. Baste with pan juices. Turn and broil for 7 minutes. (Fish should be moist but flake easily when tested with fork.) Sprinkle with parsley and serve on warmed individual serving plates.

YIELD: Serves 4

## BROILED FILLET OF WEAKFISH

Weakfish, which is rarely featured in restaurants or supermarkets, has been unduly neglected. That's a shame, because its flesh is slightly sweet and utterly delicious. It lends itself superbly to simple preparation, as you'll discover when you try this easy-to-make recipe.

2 tablespoons each dry vermouth and wine vinegar

1 tablespoon combined minced fresh parsley and dill

3 tablespoons apple juice (no sugar added)

2 cloves garlic, minced

2 shallots, minced

8 dashes ground red (cayenne) pepper

1 teaspoon dried rosemary leaves, crushed

1½ pounds fresh weakfish fillets, cut into 4 serving pieces

2 large fresh mushrooms, washed, dried, trimmed, and coarsely chopped

1 tablespoon minced sweet green pepper

1 tablespoon corn oil
Lemon wedges for garnish

1. Combine and blend first 7 listed ingredients in bowl. Wash fish and pat dry with paper toweling. Add fillets to bowl and marinate for 30 minutes at room temperature. Drain, reserving marinade.

2. Place in broiling pan. Sprinkle with mushrooms and sweet green pepper. Spoon with 2 tablespoons marinade, then dribble with corn oil. Broil 4 to 5 inches from heat for 7 minutes.

3. Spoon with balance of marinade. Return to broiler for 5 minutes. Baste with pan juices. Serve immediately on warmed individual plates, garnished with lemon wedges.

YIELD: Serves 4

## BROILED SALMON STEAKS WITH MINT

Here's a new and stimulating flavor for the king of the sea. Quickly made in your tabletop or oven broiler, it's a delicious departure from humdrum butter- and salt-broiled salmon.

### For the sauce:

½ cup fresh mint leaves, washed, dried, and minced
3 tablespoons apple cider vinegar
⅓ cup apple juice (no sugar added)
1 tablespoon honey (optional)

### For the fish:

1½ pounds fresh salmon steaks, cut into 4 serving pieces
4 teaspoons corn oil
8 dashes ground red (cayenne) pepper
2 large shallots, minced
2 large cloves garlic, minced
½ rib celery, minced
2 teaspoons minced sweet green pepper

1. Prepare the sauce the day before or 2 hours before serving. Place mint leaves and vinegar in jar. Combine apple juice and honey in saucepan. Heat until barely simmering. Pour into jar, shaking to blend.

2. Wash fish and pat dry with paper toweling. Coat on both sides with equal amounts of oil and ground red pepper. Arrange steaks on rack in broiling pan. Sprinkle with half each of shallots, garlic, celery, and green pepper. Broil 3 to 4 inches from heat for 7 minutes. Spoon each serving with 2 teaspoons mint sauce. Return to broiler for 1 minute. Turn. Sprinkle with balance of garlic and vegetables. Broil for 7 minutes. Spoon each serving with 2 teaspoons mint sauce. Return to broiler for 1 minute or until done. (Fish should flake easily when tested with fork; do not overcook.)

3. Serve immediately on warmed individual plates, with balance of mint sauce, at room temperature, in sauceboat.

YIELD: Serves 4

## BROILED SWORDFISH STEAKS

Here's how to turn a "broiling" into a "super broiling." Marinate briefly with vermouth, vinegar, herbs and spices, and broil rapidly. Enjoy then the majestic texture of this fish permeated with tongue-tingling flavors.

¼ cup each dry vermouth and wine vinegar
1 large clove garlic, minced (optional)
½ teaspoon each dried tarragon and chervil leaves, crushed
½ teaspoon each curry powder and chili con carne seasoning
4 dashes ground red (cayenne) pepper
1 small bay leaf
1½ pounds swordfish (¾ inch thick), cut into 4 serving pieces
Lemon wedges and crisp watercress sprigs for garnish

1. Make marinade by combining first 6 listed ingredients in baking dish, stirring to blend.
2. Wash fish and pat dry with paper toweling. Add to marinade, turning several times to coat. Cover and let stand at room temperature for 15 to 30 minutes. Drain, reserving marinade.
3. Arrange steaks on rack in broiling pan. Broil 4 to 5 inches from heat for 4 minutes. Spoon with marinade and turn. Broil for 4 minutes. Repeat basting and turning procedure twice more until fish is done. (Fish should be cooked through but juicy; do not overcook.)
4. Serve immediately on warmed individual plates, garnished with lemon wedges and watercress.

YIELD: Serves 4

## FLOUNDER AND RICE CASSEROLE

Flounder, one of the least flavorsome of all schools of fish, goes to the head of the class when it's flash cooked, then arranged on top of a piping hot tomato-rice casserole. As satisfying as it is delicious.

2 teaspoons each corn oil and Italian olive oil, combined, plus ¼ teaspoon for casserole

2 tablespoons each minced sweet green pepper and celery

3 cloves garlic, minced

2 large fresh mushrooms, washed, dried, trimmed, and coarsely chopped

6 dashes ground red (cayenne) pepper

½ teaspoon each curry powder (no salt or pepper added), and dried thyme leaves, crushed

¼ teaspoon ground marjoram

¾ cup uncooked rice

¼ cup dry vermouth

¼ cup Miracle Chicken Stock (page 168)

⅓ cup apple juice (no sugar added)

1 cup canned tomatoes (no salt added), chopped

Bouquet garni (made with 1 sprig each parsley and dill and 1 bay leaf tied together with white thread)

1 pound fresh flounder fillets, cut into 1-inch pieces

2 teaspoons fresh lemon juice

1. Heat half of combined oils in nonstick skillet until hot. Sauté green pepper, celery, garlic, and mushrooms over medium heat until wilted but not brown. Sprinkle with spices and dried herbs. Stir.

2. Add rice. Stir and sauté for 1 minute.

3. Add vermouth and simmer for 30 seconds.

4. Add stock, apple juice, tomatoes, and bouquet garni.

5. Bring to simmering point. Pour into lightly oiled 1½-quart casserole. Cover and bake in preheated 375°F oven for 20 minutes.

6. Wipe out skillet. Heat balance of oils (2 teaspoons) in skillet until hot. Sauté fish over high heat for 1 minute on each side. Sprinkle with lemon juice.

7. Remove casserole from oven. Uncover. With spatula, carefully place sautéed fish on top of rice. Re-cover and bake for 10 minutes.

8. Serve immediately at table directly from casserole.

YIELD: Serves 4

SERVING SUGGESTION: A crisp green salad such as watercress or arrugula makes a fine simple accompaniment to this hearty dish.

# CHICKEN

## SAVORY SAUTÉED CHICKEN

"What, chicken *again?*" is a familiar dieter's lament. That's why I've invented a wide variety of chicken dishes to replace monotony-stress with delightful surprises. Here's one. And there are more to come.

4 chicken legs with thighs (2 pounds), skinned, legs separated from thighs
About ½ teaspoon ground ginger
8 dashes ground red (cayenne) pepper
2 teaspoons each corn oil and Italian olive oil, combined
1 medium leek, white part only, well washed, dried, and coarsely chopped
3 large cloves garlic, minced
½-inch slice fresh ginger, peeled and shredded
2 large fresh mushrooms, washed, dried, trimmed, and coarsely chopped
2 tablespoons minced sweet green pepper
½ rib celery, minced
½ teaspoon each dried rosemary and thyme leaves, crushed
¼ cup dry vermouth
3 tablespoons partially thawed orange juice concentrate (no sugar added)
½ teaspoon grated orange rind, preferably from navel orange
2 tablespoons Miracle Chicken Stock (page 168; optional)

1. Wash chicken under cold running water and pat dry with paper toweling. Sprinkle and rub with ginger and ground red pepper.
2. Heat half of combined oils in well-seasoned iron skillet until hot. Turn heat down to medium. Sauté chicken until lightly browned on both sides (about 5 minutes). Transfer to bowl. Pour out any liquid in skillet.
3. Add balance of oil (2 teaspoons) to skillet. Sauté leek, garlic, ginger, mushrooms, sweet green pepper, and celery until lightly browned. Sprinkle with herbs. Stir to blend.
4. Add vermouth. Cook for 30 seconds. Add orange juice concentrate, orange rind, and stock. Bring to simmering point, spooning liquid over chicken. Cover and simmer gently over very low heat until tender, turning often (about 45 minutes). Transfer chicken to warmed serving dish. Cover to keep warm.
5. Turn up heat under skillet. Reduce liquid by half. Pour into fine sieve, pressing out juices. Pour over chicken and serve.

YIELD: Serves 4

NOTE: To keep your iron skillet well seasoned wash in soapy water (do not soak). Dry thoroughly. Rub with oil. Place skillet over medium heat for 3 minutes, then let cool. Wipe out skillet with paper toweling. Your skillet is now ready to use with a minimum amount of oil, and it will remain rust-free indefinitely.

## UNFRIED FRIED CHICKEN

Fried chicken fans—here's good news. You don't have to give up that "crisp on the outside, moist on the inside" taste you love. I've herbed and spiced a tender young chicken, coated it with healthful ingredients, and *baked* it to satisfy your demand for moistness and crispness. You have to taste it to believe it.

1 tablespoon partially thawed orange juice concentrate (no sugar added)

⅓ cup evaporated skim milk

1 broiling chicken (3 pounds), skinned, cut into eighths, wing tips removed

⅓ cup bread crumbs (salt-free)

2 tablespoons each toasted wheat germ (no sugar added) and unprocessed bran

1 teaspoon dried rosemary leaves, crushed

1 teaspoon curry powder (no salt or pepper added)

½ teaspoon cuminseed, crushed

6 dashes ground red (cayenne) pepper

1 teaspoon corn oil

1. Combine orange juice concentrate and milk in medium bowl. Blend. Wash chicken parts and dry thoroughly with paper toweling. Place chicken in bowl, turning to coat.

2. In another bowl, combine bread crumbs, wheat germ, bran, rosemary, and spices. Blend well.

3. Drain chicken. Dip each piece into crumb mixture, turning to coat. Place coated chicken on plate in one layer. Cover and refrigerate for 30 minutes.

4. Spread oil over shallow metal broiling pan. Place pan in preheated 400°F oven for 3 minutes. Remove from oven. Lay chicken in pan in one layer. Reduce oven to 375°F. Bake, uncovered, for 30 to 40 minutes, carefully turning once midway with spatula, piggybacking smaller pieces (which get done fastest) on top of larger pieces.

YIELD: Serves 4

## LEMON-LIME CHICKEN

Here's everybody's favorite, chicken breasts, briefly sautéed in herbs and corn oil, then bathed in a lemon-lime sauce. The inspiration for this slightly tart and moist chicken is Oriental, but the result is All-American.

2 whole chicken breasts, boned and skinned (1½ pounds boned weight)
½ teaspoon each dried rosemary and savory leaves, crushed
8 dashes ground red (cayenne) pepper
2 teaspoons corn oil
3 cloves garlic, minced
1 medium leek, including 2 inches of green part, well washed and minced
1 tablespoon minced sweet red pepper
½ rib celery, minced
¼ cup dry vermouth
¼ cup Miracle Chicken Stock (page 168)
½ each fresh lemon and lime, thinly sliced
2 tablespoons minced fresh parsley
2 teaspoons sweet (unsalted) 100 percent corn oil margarine

1. Wash chicken breasts under cold running water and pat dry with paper toweling. Sprinkle and rub with herbs and ground red pepper.

2. Heat oil in nonstick skillet until hot. Add chicken and brown lightly on both sides. Transfer to plate.

3. Add garlic, leek, sweet red pepper, and celery to skillet. Sauté until wilted but not brown, stirring constantly. Add vermouth. Cook for 1 minute. Add stock, lemon and lime slices, and 1 tablespoon minced parsley. Bring to simmering point.

4. Return chicken to skillet, turning to coat. Cover and simmer gently for 15 minutes, basting and turning every 5 minutes. Transfer chicken to plate. Cover to keep warm.

5. Discard lemon and lime slices. Turn heat up under skillet and reduce sauce for 3 minutes, stirring constantly. Add margarine, stirring until dissolved. Pour over chicken and serve.

YIELD: Serves 4

VARIATION: For a creamy-textured sauce, pour reduced sauce (step 5) into blender. Blend until smooth. Pour over chicken and serve.

SERVING SUGGESTION: Delicious over a bed of rice.

## CRANBERRY CHICKEN BREASTS

Take advantage of the crop of tangy, tart cranberries in December by freezing several bags (they take up so little space). Then whenever you feel the urge for an utterly unusual dish, bring them out of storage and use them in this taste-titillating recipe.

2 whole chicken breasts, boned and skinned (1½ pounds boned weight)
1 teaspoon dried rosemary leaves, crushed
8 dashes ground red (cayenne) pepper
½ teaspoon curry powder (no salt or pepper added)
1 tablespoon corn oil
½ rib celery, minced
2 large cloves garlic, minced
1 small onion, minced
2 tablespoons minced sweet red or green pepper
1 tablespoon grated carrot
1 tart crisp apple, peeled, cored, and coarsely chopped
⅓ cup Miracle Chicken Stock (page 168)
½ cup fresh cranberries
½ teaspoon ground cinnamon
¼ cup apple juice (no sugar added)

1. Wash chicken. Pat dry with paper toweling. Sprinkle and rub on both sides with rosemary, ground red pepper, and curry powder.

2. Heat oil in nonstick skillet until hot. Sauté celery, garlic, onion, sweet pepper, and carrot for 1 minute. Lay seasoned chicken on top of mixture. Sauté on both sides until lightly browned (about 8 minutes).

3. Add apple. Sauté for 1 minute. Add stock, cranberries, and cinnamon. Bring to simmering point. Turn chicken several times in liquid. Cover tightly and simmer for 15 minutes, turning once midway. Remove from heat. Let stand, covered, for 10 minutes. Transfer chicken to warmed serving plate. Cover to keep warm.

4. Add apple juice to skillet. Turn heat up and reduce cooking liquid by half, stirring constantly. Strain, pressing out juices from solids. Spoon hot sauce over chicken and serve.

YIELD: Serves 4

## SWEET AND LOVELY ROAST CHICKEN

Removing the skin *before* cooking is a must in my cuisine (about 25 percent of the chicken's fat is discarded that way). What to do with a naked bird? Bathe it in any of my many exotic marinades, prepare it following my simple directions, and enjoy chicken flavors you never dreamed could exist.

1 broiling chicken (3 pounds), skinned, wing tips removed
1 recipe Versatile Marinade (page 164)

1. Wash chicken inside and out under cold running water and pat dry with paper toweling. Place in large bowl.

2. Pour marinade over chicken, spooning some into cavity. Marinate for 1 hour at room temperature, or cover tightly and refrigerate overnight. Remove from refrigerator 1 hour before cooking.

3. Drain chicken, reserving marinade. Place chicken on rack in shallow roasting pan. Cover loosely with aluminum foil. Roast in preheated 375°F oven for 20 minutes. Uncover. Spoon with half of marinade. Re-cover and roast another 25 minutes. Pour balance of marinade over chicken. Re-cover and return to oven for 15 minutes. Baste. Roast, uncovered, for 5 minutes.

4. Cut into serving pieces and serve.

YIELD: Serves 4

VARIATION: Chicken may be cut into serving pieces, skinned, and marinated, and then broiled. Here's how: Drain chicken, reserving marinade. Preheat broiler. Set rack in high position. Lay chicken on rack and broil for 7 minutes. Turn. Spoon with marinade and broil for 7 minutes. Turn and brush again, then continue to broil, turning and brushing twice more at 7-minute intervals, until done (total cooking time is 35 minutes). Should smaller parts be done before rest of bird, tuck them under larger pieces to keep warm.

## EASY-TO-MAKE INDIAN-STYLE ROAST CHICKEN

If you've shied away from Indian food, it's high time you put a little adventure into your life. This mild-tasting chicken, tenderly marinated with the spices of India, could be your introduction to a new exciting world of flavors. You'll love it!

1 tablespoon wine vinegar
1 tablespoon corn oil
¼ cup fresh orange juice
½ cup plain low-fat yogurt
3 large cloves garlic, minced
1 teaspoon each cuminseed, crushed, and curry powder (no salt or pepper added)
⅛ teaspoon ground red (cayenne) pepper
½ teaspoon each ground cinnamon and ginger
1 broiling chicken (3 pounds), skinned, wing tips removed

1. Combine all ingredients except chicken in large bowl. Beat with whisk to blend.

2. Wash chicken inside and out under cold running water. Dry thoroughly with paper toweling. Add chicken to bowl, turning to coat, and spooning cavity with marinade. Let stand for 1 hour, or cover and refrigerate overnight.

3. Follow steps 3 and 4 in recipe for Sweet and Lovely Roast Chicken (page 134) to complete recipe, including variation.

YIELD: Serves 4

## SKILLET CHICKEN DINNER

Stock, herbs, spices, and a suggestion of orange combined with chicken and potatoes will bring out the ooohs and aaahs your family has been storing up for that special dish. For a light but satisfying repast, just precede with a simple salad.

1 whole chicken breast, boned and skinned (1½ pounds boned weight), cut into 4 pieces
2 small chicken legs with thighs, skinned (about 1 pound), legs separated from thighs
½ teaspoon each dried savory and marjoram leaves, crushed
⅛ teaspoon ground red (cayenne) pepper
4 teaspoons corn oil
3 large cloves garlic, minced
1 small onion, minced
1 tablespoon minced sweet red pepper
2 teaspoons peeled and minced fresh ginger
2 tablespoons Miracle Chicken Stock (page 168)
¼ cup dry vermouth
1 teaspoon chili con carne seasoning (no salt or pepper added)
4 small red-skinned potatoes (about ½ pound), peeled and cut into 1-inch cubes
1 navel orange, peeled and cut into 1-inch chunks
2 tablespoons minced fresh parsley

1. Wash chicken under cold running water and pat dry with paper toweling. Sprinkle and rub with dried herbs and ground red pepper.

2. Heat 3 teaspoons oil in nonstick skillet until hot. Add chicken and brown lightly on both sides. Transfer to dish.

3. Heat balance of oil (1 teaspoon) until hot. Add garlic, onion, sweet red pepper, and ginger. Sauté until lightly browned.

4. Combine stock, vermouth, and chili con carne seasoning. Add to skillet, stirring to blend. Bring to simmering point. Return chicken to skillet. Cover and simmer gently for 10 minutes.

5. Add potatoes and orange, making sure they're immersed in liquid. Bring to simmering point. Re-cover and simmer for 15 minutes. Uncover and cook over medium-high heat until most of liquid is reduced and chicken legs are tender.

6. Transfer chicken to warmed serving plate. Spoon with reduced sauce. Sprinkle with parsley and serve.

YIELD: Serves 4

SERVING SUGGESTION: Simple-to-make Watercress-Mushroom Salad (page 188) is the only accompaniment you'll need with this dish.

## QUICK AND EASY MOIST ORANGE CHICKEN

Only eight ingredients combine to make this simplest of chicken dishes a smashing success. It's a weekly favorite in our household.

1 broiling chicken (3 pounds), skinned, wing tips removed
4 ounces partially thawed frozen orange juice concentrate (no sugar added)
1 tablespoon fresh lime juice
2 teaspoons chili con carne seasoning (no salt or pepper added)
4 dashes ground cloves
8 dashes ground red (cayenne) pepper
3 large cloves garlic, minced
¼ cup loosely packed minced fresh mint or basil

1. Wash chicken inside and out under cold running water and pat dry with paper toweling. Place in bowl.

2. Prepare basting sauce by combining balance of ingredients, except fresh mint or basil, in jar and shaking well. Pour over chicken, spooning some into cavity. Stand chicken upright and drain, reserving basting sauce.

3. Place chicken on rack in shallow roasting pan. Cover loosely with aluminum foil. Roast in preheated 375°F oven for 20 minutes. Uncover. Spoon with half of basting sauce. Re-cover and roast another 25 minutes. Pour balance of basting sauce over chicken. Re-cover and return to oven for 10 minutes. Baste with pan juices. Roast, uncovered, for 5 minutes.

4. Cut chicken into serving pieces. Arrange on platter. Sprinkle with fresh mint or basil and serve.

YIELD: Serves 4

VARIATION: For a fabulous outdoor grill, cut raw chicken into serving pieces and marinate in basting sauce for 1 hour. Drain chicken. Grill, turning and basting frequently with basting sauce. Sprinkle finished chicken with fresh mint and serve.

NOTE: *Fresh* herbs make this recipe outstanding. Do not substitute dried herbs. If fresh mint or basil is not available, substitute fresh tarragon, rosemary, or dill.

# VEGETABLES, RICE, AND PASTA

## SAUTÉED GREEN BEANS

Tender green beans, an excellent source of fiber, is—alas!—a humdrum vegetable as it comes to your kitchen. But herbed, spiced, and bathed in a light savory sauce, it's transformed into a sophisticated offering that will enhance just about any main course.

1 pound fresh green beans, washed, each bean cut in half
1 tablespoon corn oil
2 cloves garlic, minced
2 shallots, minced
2 large fresh mushrooms, washed, dried, trimmed, and thinly sliced
1 teaspoon peeled and minced fresh ginger
1 teaspoon each dried rosemary leaves, crushed, and minced fresh dill
8 dashes ground red (cayenne) pepper
1 teaspoon tomato paste (no salt added)
3 tablespoons Miracle Chicken Stock (page 168)
3 tablespoons evaporated skim milk

1. Drop beans into pot of rapidly boiling water. Boil until almost tender (cooking time will vary with thickness and age of bean). Drain.

2. Heat oil in nonstick skillet until hot. Sauté garlic, shallots, mushrooms, and ginger until just wilted (do not brown), stirring constantly. Add green beans, stirring to coat. Sauté for 1 minute over medium-high heat. Sprinkle with herbs and ground red pepper.

3. Combine tomato paste and chicken stock. Pour into skillet. Stir and cook ingredients only until well heated.

4. Remove from heat. Stir in milk. Serve immediately.

YIELD: Serves 4

VARIATIONS:

1. For added crunchiness and color, add in step two ½ sweet red pepper, cut into ⅜-inch slivers.

2. Substitute cut, slightly undercooked fresh asparagus for green beans, taking care not to break tips when stirring.

## SCRUMPTIOUS POTATO PANCAKES

Potato pancakes rise to new heights in this low-calorie, low-fat version. Delicately seasoned with herbs and spices, and rapidly sautéed to a crisp golden brown, they should—just as rapidly—become a favorite in your household.

3 tablespoons unbleached flour
1¼ teaspoons low-sodium baking powder
½ teaspoon ground ginger
8 dashes ground red (cayenne) pepper
¼ teaspoon dried thyme leaves, crushed
3 medium baking potatoes, peeled
1 medium carrot, peeled
½ teaspoon fresh lemon juice
1 egg (use ½ of yolk and all of white)
2 cloves garlic, minced
1 large shallot or scallion, minced
¼ cup loosely packed minced fresh basil (see note)
1 tablespoon plain low-fat yogurt, plus more, if desired, for garnish
1 teaspoon corn oil, for skillet
Minced fresh parsley or dill (optional)

1. Combine flour, baking powder, ginger, ground red pepper, and thyme in bowl. Stir to blend. Set aside.

2. Grate potatoes into another bowl. Press mixture with spoon against sides of bowl to drain off excess water.

Grate carrot into mixture. Stir in lemon juice.

3. Combine egg, garlic, and shallot in cup. Beat with fork to blend. Stir into potato mixture. Add basil and dry ingredients. Blend. Fold in yogurt.

4. Brush skillet with small amount of the oil; heat until hot. Sauté 4 pancakes at a time, using 1 tablespoon of batter for each pancake, then flattening with spoon. Sauté until brown and crispy on both sides (do not overcook). Brush skillet with more oil and repeat process twice more. (Cooked pancakes may be kept warm in 350°F oven until all 12 have been prepared. Do not stack.)

5. Serve immediately, plain, or with a dollop of low-fat plain yogurt and a sprinkling of minced fresh parsley or dill.

YIELD: 12 pancakes; serves 6 as a side dish, 3 as a luncheon dish.

NOTE: If fresh basil isn't available, try crisp watercress leaves, minced.

## SAUTÉED VEGETABLES WITH APPLES

No plain mashed potatoes tonight! Here potatoes are combined with apples and colorful red pepper to create a fabulous new dish. Slightly tart, it's a wonderful accompaniment to meat and poultry dishes.

2 medium potatoes (about 1¼ pounds), peeled and cut into ⅜-inch slices

1 medium sweet red pepper, seeded and cut into ½-inch slices

1 tablespoon corn oil

2 medium onions, peeled, cut into ¼-inch slices

2 large shallots, minced

2 tart apples, peeled, cored, cut into ⅜-inch slices

8 dashes ground red (cayenne) pepper

¼ teaspoon ground cinnamon

½ teaspoon dried rosemary leaves, crushed

2 tablespoons each Miracle Chicken Stock (page 168) and apple juice, no sugar added

1 tablespoon minced fresh parsley

1. Cook potatoes in pot of rapidly boiling water for 8 minutes. Drain and set aside.

2. Blanch seeded whole sweet red pepper by dropping into rapidly boiling water for 1 minute. Drain, cut, and set aside.

3. Heat oil in nonstick skillet until hot. Add onions and shallots. Sauté until wilted but not brown. Add potatoes, sweet red pepper, and apples. Sprinkle with spices and rosemary. Stir and sauté over medium-high heat until all ingredients are heated through.

4. Add stock and apple juice. Sauté vegetables for 2 minutes longer, stirring constantly. Turn onto warmed serving plate, sprinkle with parsley, and serve.

YIELD: Serves 4

NOTE: If you're the proud possessor of a wok, try this recipe in that wonder-working utensil. Heat wok for 1½ minutes, pour oil around rim, and continue with recipe. Vegetables will be crispier, the flavor slightly different—and you'll experience a refreshing new taste.

## PRETTY POTATOES À L'ORANGE

There's nothing more satisfying when you're hungry than potatoes. But all you're allowed on most diets that *do* allow potatoes are the baked and boiled varieties. Great! But not day after day after day. Here's a zestful new-style mashed potato with a soufflé-like consistency that will delight you. Easy to prepare, too.

1½ pounds potatoes, peeled, cubed, and cooked
1 tablespoon corn oil
1 large clove garlic, minced
2 large shallots, minced
1 medium onion or 1 large green onion, minced
2 tablespoons minced fresh tarragon, rosemary, or dill
½ teaspoon curry powder (no salt or pepper added)
4 dashes ground red (cayenne) pepper
1 teaspoon grated orange rind, preferably from navel orange
3 tablespoons plain low-fat yogurt
½ teaspoon sweet (unsalted) 100 percent corn oil margarine, for crocks

1. Mash potatoes while still warm. Place in bowl.
2. Heat oil in nonstick skillet until hot. Add garlic, shallots, and onion. Sauté briefly until wilted. Add to bowl with potatoes. Blend.
3. Add herbs, spices, and orange rind. Blend. Stir in yogurt.
4. Grease 4 individual ovenproof crocks with margarine. Fill with potatoes. Bake in preheated 425°F oven for 20 minutes. (Mixture will puff up and tops will be lightly browned.) Serve immediately.

YIELD: Serves 4

VARIATION: Cut 2 large navel oranges in half. Cut out and reserve several segments for garnish and the balance for salads; reserve shells. Pile mashed potatoes into orange shells. Bake until heated through in preheated 425°F oven (15 to 20 minutes). Garnish with sliced orange segments and serve.

## STIR-FRIED BROCCOLI AND PEPPERS

I believe every dieter should make a modest investment in a wok. It's the simplest and most expedient way of preparing food without excess oil or seasonings. Vegetables come to the table crunchy and naturally delicious, and they retain almost all of their precious nutrients. Prepare a wokful of this basic recipe and quickly revel in a new taste experience. (See *Francine Prince's New Gourmet Recipes for Dieters* for explicit instructions and more recipes for low-calorie cooking with a wok.)

Flowerets from 2 stalks broccoli (about 4 cups)
1 medium sweet red pepper, seeded and cut into ½-inch slices
1 tablespoon corn oil
1 tablespoon peeled and shredded fresh ginger
2 large cloves garlic, minced
1 teaspoon dried rosemary leaves, crushed
⅛ teaspoon ground red (cayenne) pepper
¼ cup Miracle Chicken Stock (page 168)
1 tablespoon medium-dry sherry

1. Parboil broccoli and sweet red pepper by dropping into rapidly boiling water for 1 minute. Drain in colander. Place colander under cold running water to stop cooking action. Set aside.

2. Heat wok for 1½ minutes over high heat. Pour oil around rim of wok. Add ginger and garlic. Stir-fry for 15 seconds. Add broccoli and sweet red pepper. Sprinkle with rosemary and ground red pepper and stir-fry for 1 minute.

3. Combine stock and sherry. Pour around rim of wok. Stir. Cover and cook over medium heat for 1½ minutes. Serve immediately.

YIELD: Serves 4

VARIATIONS:

1. Substitute ¼ cup apple juice (no sugar added) for stock and substitute 2 tablespoons dry vermouth for sherry.

2. One pound tender green beans may be prepared in the same fashion as broccoli. Parboil for 4 to 7 minutes, depending upon maturity of beans, adding sweet red pepper to green beans 1 minute before completion of prescribed cooking time.

3. Add in step two ½ teaspoon smoked yeast (available in health food stores) for a slightly bacon-y flavor.

## POTATO-CARROT MEDLEY

The busy working dieter can prepare these marriageable vegetables quickly the night before, refrigerate them, and complete the recipe in minutes just before dinnertime. It's so quick and easy, why would you want to settle for prepared commercial vegetables ever again?

¾ pound medium red-skinned potatoes, washed

3 medium carrots, peeled and cut into ½-inch matchstick-shaped pieces

1 tablespoon corn oil

2 large cloves garlic, minced

2 large shallots, minced

¾ teaspoon each cuminseed, crushed, and ground ginger

8 dashes ground red (cayenne) pepper

1 tablespoon each minced fresh parsley and dill, combined

1. Cook potatoes and carrots together in rapidly boiling water until tender (about 15 minutes). Drain. Let cool to room temperature. Peel potatoes. Set aside.

2. Heat oil in nonstick skillet until hot. Sauté garlic and shallots over medium heat for 1 minute. Add potatoes and carrots. Sauté until heated through. Sprinkle with spices. Sauté for 5 minutes, turning often.

3. Turn into serving dish. Sprinkle with minced parsley and dill and serve.

YIELD: Serves 4

VARIATIONS: Try the same basic recipe with the following parboiled vegetable combinations: broccoli and carrots, cabbage and carrots, potatoes and small white onions, green beans and sweet red peppers, and cauliflower and snow peas.

## TURNIP-LEEK PURÉE

Turnips are rarely found in the recipes of gourmet chefs. But my vegetable bin is never without them. They contribute so much flavor to soups and stocks. Here, white turnip combined with leek, herbs, and spices becomes a culinary delight that will perk up any simple meat, fish, or poultry dish.

2 teaspoons corn oil

1½ cups diced leek, white part and 1 inch of green part, well washed (about 4 leeks)

1 pound white turnip, peeled and cut into ½-inch cubes

¾ cup Miracle Chicken Stock (page 168)

¼ cup dry vermouth

½ cup apple juice (no sugar added)

1 tablespoon combined minced fresh parsley and dill

½ teaspoon dried tarragon leaves, crushed

½ teaspoon ground coriander

⅛ teaspoon ground red (cayenne) pepper

1. Heat oil in nonstick skillet until hot. Sauté leeks for 2 minutes, taking care they do not brown. Add turnip and sauté for 2 minutes.

2. Add stock, vermouth, apple juice, herbs, and spices. Bring to simmering point. Cover and simmer until turnip is tender but not oversoft (about 45 minutes; you will notice that most of the liquid will have evaporated at the end of cooking time). Remove from heat. Let stand, covered, for 10 minutes.

3. Turn into food processor workbowl (see note below) and process for 10 seconds. Stop machine. Scrape down sides of workbowl. Turn processor on/off several times until you reach desired consistency. (Finished purée should be textured and not oversmooth.)

4. Return mixture to skillet and reheat until heated through. Serve immediately.

YIELD: Serves 4

NOTE: Sautéed ingredients may be turned into a food mill and puréed to desired texture.

## DELICIOUS TOFU CASSEROLE

Hooray for tofu! It's a high-protein substitute for meat, fish, and poultry—low in fat and cholesterol; and half a pound of it has only 184 calories! Its own flavor is undistinguishable—but, oh, how it soaks up a cornucopia of flavors! Rush out to your oriental market or regular supermarket for your tofu cakes, then transform them into this spectacularly flavorsome casserole.

2 tofu cakes (each 3 inches square)
2 teaspoons each corn oil and Italian olive oil, combined
1 medium sweet green pepper, seeded and minced
3 medium onions, minced
3 large cloves garlic, minced
2 whole scallions, minced
1 teaspoon peeled and minced fresh ginger
4 large fresh mushrooms, washed, dried, trimmed, and thinly sliced
2 tablespoons minced fresh parsley
¼ cup dry vermouth
2 tablespoons apple juice (no sugar added)
1 cup canned tomatoes (no salt added), chopped
2 teaspoons tomato paste (no salt added)
½ teaspoon each dried thyme and marjoram leaves, crushed
1 teaspoon chili con carne seasoning (no salt or pepper added)
3 dashes ground red (cayenne) pepper (optional)
1 teaspoon yellow cornmeal

1. Lay tofu cakes on doubled sheets of paper toweling. Let drain, turning twice. Cut into ½-inch slices. Set aside.

2. Heat combined oils in large nonstick skillet until hot. Sauté green pepper, onions, garlic, scallions, and ginger until softened (about 5 minutes), stirring constantly. Add mushrooms. Sauté for 2 minutes, taking care that ingredients do not brown. Sprinkle with parsley. Stir.

3. Add vermouth and apple juice. Cook for 1 minute. Add balance of ingredients (except for reserved tofu), stirring to combine. Reduce heat to simmering. Cook, uncovered, for 3 minutes. Mixture will be smooth and thick.

4. Pour half of mixture into a 10 × 6-inch baking dish or pan. Arrange tofu over mixture, overlapping slices. Cover with remaining mixture, smoothing out into corners with spoon. Bake, uncovered, in preheated 350°F oven until bubbly and tofu is heated through (about 20 minutes).

YIELD: Serves 4

VARIATIONS:

1. In step 4, sprinkle sauce with ½ teaspoon no-fat Sap Sago cheese. Cover with tofu slices. Add balance of sauce. Sprinkle with another ½ teaspoon no-fat Sap Sago.

2. Substitute ¼ cup Miracle Chicken Stock (page 168) for vermouth and add 1 tablespoon apple cider vinegar to recipe.

NOTE: Entire dish may be prepared well ahead of time and refrigerated. Remove from refrigerator 30 minutes before baking.

# PASTA

Pasta while you're dieting? Of course! It's high in protein and fiber, low in fat and cholesterol, and the right kind is salt free. Calorie count, even with my sauce for pasta lovers, is only 300 to 325 per portion. Here are three examples of how delicious slimming pasta dishes can taste. I call the first of these Prego Linguine, because in Italy *prego* means all sorts of happy things including "thank you," and "please," and "have a good day." Have a happy meal every time you serve it—and all my other pasta dishes.

## PREGO LINGUINE

2 teaspoons each corn oil and Italian olive oil, combined

1 rib celery, minced

3 large cloves garlic, minced

2 medium onions, minced

1 tablespoon peeled and shredded fresh ginger

1 medium sweet green pepper, seeded and minced

¼ pound fresh mushrooms, washed, dried, trimmed, and sliced

2 teaspoons dried rosemary leaves, crushed

8 dashes ground red (cayenne) pepper

¼ cup each dry vermouth, Miracle Chicken Stock (page 168), and apple juice (no sugar added)

1 cup canned tomatoes (no salt added), chopped

1 tablespoon tomato paste (no salt added)

½ cup tomato purée (no salt added)

Bouquet garni (3 sprigs fresh parsley, 1 bay leaf, tied together with white thread)

¾ pound whole-wheat or enriched linguine (no salt added)

1. Heat half of combined oils in well-seasoned iron skillet (see note 2) until hot but not smoking. Add celery, garlic, onions, ginger, and sweet green pepper. Sauté over medium heat until wilted but not brown, stirring often so that ingredients do not stick. Push mixture to side of skillet. Add balance of oil (2 teaspoons) to skillet and sauté mushrooms for 3 minutes, stirring constantly. Combine ingredients in skillet. Sprinkle with rosemary and ground red pepper and stir.

2. Add vermouth, stock, and apple juice. Bring to simmering point.

3. Add tomatoes, tomato paste, tomato purée, and bouquet garni. Stir. Bring to simmering point. Reduce heat, cover, and simmer gently for 1 hour, stirring 4 times. Turn off heat. Let stand, covered, while preparing linguine.

4. Bring large pot of water to rolling boil. Add linguine. Bring to boiling point again and boil for 8 to 10 minutes, stirring often (do not overcook). Drain. Transfer to large serving bowl.

5. Remove bouquet garni from sauce. Pour hot sauce over linguine. With 2 large spoons, combine sauce briefly with pasta and serve.

YIELD: Serves 6

NOTES:

1. To serve 4, prepare 8 ounces linguine, use two thirds of the sauce, and freeze balance of sauce for another meal for 2.

2. For directions on how to prepare a well-seasoned iron skillet, see Note for Savory Sautéed Chicken (page 130).

## PASTA SHELLS WITH SHRIMP

1 recipe Prego Linguine (page 146;
   substitute 8 ounces whole-wheat or
   enriched pasta shells [no salt added]
   for linguine)
2 teaspoons corn oil
2 tablespoons minced shallots
½ pound medium shrimp, peeled and
   deveined, cut into ½-inch pieces,
   well dried
1 tablespoon minced fresh parsley

1. Prepare sauce and pasta according to directions given for Prego Linguine. Pasta will be al dente (firm textured). Combine sauce and pasta in pot. Cover to keep warm.

2. Heat oil in nonstick skillet until hot. Spread shallots across skillet. Sauté for 30 seconds. Lay shrimps on top of shallots. Sauté on one side until shrimp turn pink (about 1½ minutes). Turn and sauté until pink on second side (do not overcook).

3. Pour pasta with sauce into serving bowl. With spoon, arrange cooked shrimp and shallots over pasta. Sprinkle with parsley and serve immediately.

YIELD: Serves 4

## PIQUANT MACARONI

2 teaspoons each corn oil and Italian olive oil, combined

1 medium sweet green pepper, seeded and cut into ¼-inch slivers

4 cloves garlic, minced

4 shallots, minced

1 rib celery, minced

2 large fresh mushrooms, washed, dried, trimmed, and thinly sliced (optional)

¾ teaspoon each dried rosemary and thyme leaves, crushed

8 dashes ground red (cayenne) pepper

½ teaspoon curry powder (no salt or pepper added)

¼ cup dry vermouth

2 cups canned tomatoes (no salt added), chopped

4 teaspoons tomato paste (no salt added)

⅓ cup tomato purée (no salt added)

¼ cup loosely packed minced fresh mint leaves, washed and dried

¾ pound whole-wheat or enriched elbow macaroni (no salt added)

2 tablespoons minced fresh parsley

1. Heat oil in well-seasoned iron skillet (see note 2 below) until hot. Sauté green pepper, garlic, shallots, celery, and mushrooms until lightly browned, stirring often so that ingredients don't stick to skillet. Sprinkle with dried herbs and spices. Stir to blend.

2. Add vermouth. Stir and cook for 1 minute.

3. Combine tomatoes, tomato paste, and tomato purée. Add to skillet. Bring to simmering point. Sprinkle with mint. Lower heat to simmering. Cover and simmer for 1 hour, stirring 4 times. Let stand, covered, while preparing macaroni.

4. Bring pot of water to rolling boil. Add macaroni and cook for 8 to 10 minutes, stirring often. (Macaroni will be al dente; cook a minute or two longer, if desired.) Drain.

5. Transfer to warmed serving bowl. Pour hot sauce over macaroni. Sprinkle with parsley and serve.

YIELD: Serves 6

VARIATION: Serve with no-fat Sap Sago cheese on the side, if desired.

NOTES:

1. To serve 4, prepare 8 ounces macaroni, use two thirds of sauce, and freeze balance of sauce for another meal for 2.

2. For directions on how to prepare a well-seasoned iron skillet, see note for Savory Sautéed Chicken on page 130.

## BROWN RICE WITH LEEK

Brown rice or white? Brown rice has the edge in fiber, but enriched rice is equally as nutritious. The following two recipes give you a chance to enjoy a quality each variety possesses—the capability of marrying with a variety of foods and flavors to produce a dish more delicious than the sum of its parts.

1½ cups cooked brown rice
1 tablespoon wine vinegar
1 tablespoon corn oil
1 medium leek, white part only, well washed and minced
2 cloves garlic, minced
½ sweet red pepper, seeded and cut into ¼-inch slivers
4 large fresh mushrooms, washed, dried, trimmed, and thinly sliced
8 dashes ground red (cayenne) pepper
½ teaspoon dried chervil leaves, crushed
2 tablespoons Miracle Chicken Stock (page 168)
¼ cup minced fresh basil or 2 tablespoons minced fresh tarragon, rosemary, or dill

1. Place cooked rice in bowl. Sprinkle with vinegar. Stir to coat. Cover and let stand for 30 minutes before continuing with recipe. (May be refrigerated and recipe completed next day.)

2. Heat oil in nonstick skillet until hot. Sauté leek, garlic, sweet pepper, and mushrooms until wilted. Add rice, sprinkle with ground red pepper and chervil, and sauté until rice is heated through.

3. Stir in stock and basil. Cook for 30 seconds. Turn into warmed serving dish and serve immediately.

YIELD: Serves 4

VARIATION: For a slightly sweet rice, substitute apple juice (no sugar added) for stock.

## ORANGE RICE

¾ cup uncooked brown rice
¾ cup each water and Miracle Chicken Stock (page 168)
3 tablespoons partially thawed orange juice concentrate (no sugar added)
2 teaspoons corn oil
2 cloves garlic, minced
1 large shallot, minced
4 large fresh mushrooms, washed, dried, trimmed, and sliced
¼ cup minced fresh basil or 2 tablespoons minced fresh tarragon, rosemary, mint, or dill
½ teaspoon curry powder (no salt or pepper added)
½ teaspoon grated orange rind, preferably from navel orange

1. Wash and drain rice. Place in saucepan together with water and stock. Soak for 30 minutes.

2. Add orange juice concentrate. Bring to rolling boil. Reduce heat and simmer, uncovered, until tender (about 25 minutes; all liquid will be absorbed. Add a little more water, if necessary, to complete cooking time). Set aside.

3. Heat oil in nonstick skillet until hot. Sauté garlic, shallot, and mushrooms over medium-high heat until lightly browned. Add rice and stir to blend.

4. Sprinkle with basil, curry powder, and orange rind. Toss to blend. Serve immediately.

YIELD: Serves 4

# BREADS

### BEGINNER'S LOAF

If you've never baked before, this is a seductive way to start. The hand kneading is so easy it's pure joy, and the bread is so delightfully different from anything you can buy in a store that once you taste it you'll be hooked on breadmaking for life. Advice to bread connoisseurs: Don't pass this one by because it's for beginners. Apple juice, sweet spices, and orange rind impart a touch of sweetness that's as original as it is refreshing.

1 tablespoon dry yeast or 1 premeasured package
⅓ cup warm water (105° to 115°F)
3 teaspoons honey
½ cup apple juice (no sugar added)
1 tablespoon corn oil plus ¼ teaspoon for rising bowl
¼ teaspoon ground cloves
½ teaspoon each anise seeds, crushed, and ground cinnamon
1 teaspoon grated orange rind, preferably from navel orange
¾ cup evaporated skim milk, room temperature
1 cup unbleached flour
1 tablespoon toasted wheat germ (no sugar added)
2¼ cups whole-wheat flour
¼ teaspoon sweet (unsalted) 100 percent corn oil margarine, for pan

1. Combine yeast with water and 1 teaspoon honey in large mixing bowl. Beat with fork to blend. Let stand for 7 minutes. (Mixture will puff up.)

2. Combine apple juice, balance of honey (two teaspoons), oil, spices, and orange rind in saucepan. Heat slowly until warm (105° to 115°F). Stir in milk. Pour over puffed-up yeast mixture and stir with wooden spoon.

3. Add all of unbleached flour, the wheat germ, and 1 cup whole-wheat flour. Beat with wooden spoon for 1 minute.

4. Add all but ⅛ cup of balance of whole-wheat flour, ¼ cup at a time, beating with wooden spoon after each addition. When dough becomes too difficult to handle with spoon, scoop up, turn onto lightly whole-wheat–floured board, and knead until smooth and elastic to the touch (see note, page 153, for Best-Ever French Bread). Add only enough of balance of flour to make a nonsticky dough. Shape into ball.

5. Fill fairly straight-sided rising bowl with hot water. Pour out and dry. Lightly oil. Drop dough into bowl. Cover tightly with plastic wrap and let rise at room temperature (70° to 80°F) until doubled in bulk (about 1½ hours).

6. Punch dough down. Turn onto board and knead for 1 minute. Cover with plastic wrap and let rest for 5 minutes. To shape loaf, roll dough out into 12 × 9-inch rectangle. Starting at short end, roll up tightly, tucking in sides and pressing seam to hold. Place, seam down, on a lightly margarine-greased 9½ × 6 × 2½-inch loaf pan. Cover with plastic wrap and let rise until doubled in bulk (about 1¼ hours; dough should rise above sides of pan).

7. Bake in preheated 375°F oven for 40 minutes. Remove loaf from pan and place back in oven, directly on rack. Bake for 5 minutes. Remove from oven and cool thoroughly on rack before slicing.

YIELD: 1 large loaf; 24 slices (⅜ inch each)

VARIATION: In step 3, add 1 tablespoon unprocessed bran and reduce unbleached flour by 1 tablespoon.

## BEST-EVER FRENCH BREAD

What's all this about the mystique of breadmaking? Millions of people have been making bread for thousands of years. And so can you—when you follow my simple and explicit instructions. Try your hand with this crunchy, light French bread, enriched with wheat germ, bran, and dark flour and sweetened with fruit juice. I've included three methods in this recipe (ingredients have been rearranged in the second and third methods). You'll find each method ever so easy to follow, and you'll produce—well—the best French bread you've ever tasted.

### First Method: By Hand

2½ teaspoons dry yeast
½ teaspoon honey
¼ cup warm water (105° to 115°F)
½ cup each apple juice (no sugar added) and water
1 teaspoon grated orange rind, preferably from navel orange
¼ cup whole-wheat flour
3 to 3¼ cups unbleached flour
5½ teaspoons toasted wheat germ (no sugar added)
2 teaspoons ground coriander
1 teaspoon anise seed, crushed
¼ teaspoon corn oil, for rising bowl
½ teaspoon sweet (unsalted) 100 percent corn oil margarine, for pans and waxed paper
1 egg white beaten with 1 tablespoon water
1 tablespoon sesame seeds (optional)

1. Combine yeast, honey, and ¼ cup water in large mixing bowl. Beat with fork to dissolve. Let stand for 10 minutes. (Mixture will puff up.)
2. Combine apple juice, water, and orange rind in saucepan. Heat until warm (105° to 115°F; take care that liquid is not overheated or yeast will become inactive). Pour into yeast mixture and stir.
3. Combine whole-wheat flour, 3 cups unbleached flour, wheat germ, coriander, and anise seed in bowl. Stir to blend. Add half of mixture to liquid mixture (step 2). Beat with wooden spoon until flour is absorbed. Add balance of flour mixture, a little at a time, beating with wooden spoon after each addition. When dough becomes too difficult to handle with spoon, scoop up, and turn onto lightly floured board, and knead, adding balance of flour (¼ cup) if necessary to make a smooth, elastic, and nonsticky dough (see note for kneading instructions).
4. Shape dough into ball. Drop into a lightly oiled, fairly straight-sided bowl, turning to coat. Cover tightly with plastic wrap. Let rise at room temperature (70° to 80°F) until more than doubled in bulk (1½ to 2 hours).
5. Punch dough down. Transfer to very lightly floured board and knead briefly, pressing out bubbles. Cover with waxed paper and let dough rest for 3 minutes.
6. Divide dough in half and roll each piece into a slender loaf 12 inches long. Grease two 14-inch French loaf pans with small amount of margarine. Lay loaves in pans. With serrated knife, slash each loaf diagonally 4 times. Brush with egg white mixture. Lightly grease a large sheet of waxed paper with remaining margarine. Place waxed paper,

greased side down, over pans, tucking in ends of paper to prevent dough from drying out. Let rise at room temperature until doubled in bulk (about 1½ hours).

7. Gently remove waxed paper. Brush again with egg white mixture. Sprinkle with sesame seeds. Bake in preheated 425° oven for 15 minutes. Reduce heat to 375°F and bake for 15 to 20 minutes. Finished loaves should be crisp and golden brown. Slide bread out of pans. Tap bottom of loaves with knuckles. If you hear a hollow sound, the bread is done. If not, place loaves back in oven directly on rack and bake for an additional 5 minutes.

8. Remove from oven. Let bread cool thoroughly on rack (you'll hear it crackle as it cools) before slicing.

YIELD: 2 loaves; 17 to 18 slices (1 inch each) per loaf

NOTE: Here's how to knead: Shape dough into rough ball. Flatten with heel of your hand. Fold dough over toward you. Push down and then forward with heel of your hand. Make a quarter turn. Repeat folding, pushing, and turning until texture of dough becomes smooth and elastic and dough can easily be shaped into ball. Kneading rhythmically for 7 to 10 minutes should do it. Dough must be well kneaded to develop the gluten in the flour that permits the dough to rise. The time for hand kneading varies with your adeptness in handling the dough.

**SECOND METHOD:** *Standard Size Food Processor*

2½ teaspoons dry yeast
½ teaspoon honey
¼ cup warm water (105° to 115°F)
3 to 3¼ cups unbleached flour
¼ cup whole-wheat flour
5½ teaspoons toasted wheat germ (no sugar added)
2 teaspoons ground coriander
1 teaspoon anise seed, crushed
½ cup each apple juice (no sugar added) and water
1 teaspoon grated orange rind, preferably from navel orange
1 egg white beaten with 1 tablespoon water
¼ teaspoon corn oil, for rising bowl
½ teaspoon sweet (unsalted) 100 percent corn oil margarine, for pans and waxed paper
1 tablespoon sesame seeds

1. Combine yeast, honey, and ¼ cup warm water in cup. Beat with fork to dissolve. Let stand for 10 minutes. (Mixture will puff up.)

2. Fit food processor with steel blade. Combine 3 cups unbleached flour, all of whole-wheat flour, wheat germ, coriander, and anise seed in work bowl. Process on/off 3 times. Pour yeast mixture over flour. Process on/off 4 times.

3. Combine apple juice, water, and orange rind in saucepan and heat until warm (105° to 115°F). With processor on, slowly pour warmed liquid through feed tube. (Dough will form into a ball as soon as all liquid is absorbed.) Process for 5 seconds. Remove cover. If dough is sticky, add balance of flour (¼ cup) and process for 10 seconds. Turn dough onto board and knead by hand for 1 minute.

4. To complete recipe, follow steps 4 through 8 in instructions given for First Method.

## THIRD METHOD: *Large Food Processor*

1 tablespoon dry yeast or 1 pre-measured package
1 teaspoon honey
¼ cup warm water (105° to 115°F)
6 to 6¼ cups unbleached flour
½ cup whole-wheat flour
3 tablespoons toasted wheat germ (no sugar added)
1 tablespoon ground coriander
1 teaspoon anise seed, crushed
1 cup each apple juice (no sugar added) and water
2 teaspoons grated orange rind, preferably from navel orange
1 egg white beaten with 1 tablespoon water
¼ teaspoon corn oil, for rising bowl
¾ teaspoon sweet (unsalted) 100 percent corn oil margarine, for pans and waxed paper
2 tablespoons sesame seeds

1. Follow step 1 in recipe for Second Method.

2. Fit large food processor with plastic blade. Combine 4 cups unbleached flour, all of whole wheat flour, wheat germ, coriander, and anise seed in large workbowl. Process on/off 6 times. With processor on, pour yeast mixture through feed tube. Process for ten seconds.

3. Combine apple juice, water, and orange rind in saucepan. Heat until warm (90° to 100°F). With processor on, slowly pour warmed liquid through feed tube. Stop machine. Add 2 cups unbleached flour. Process on/off twice. Then process for 10 seconds. Turn dough onto lightly floured board and knead by hand for 2 minutes.

4. To complete recipe, follow steps 4 through 8 in instructions given for First Method.

YIELD: 4 loaves; 17 to 18 slices (1 inch each) per loaf

VARIATION: Add 2 tablespoons un-processed bran to recipe and reduce amount of unbleached flour by 3 tablespoons.

NOTE: For further instructions on bread-making, including the use of a dough hook, see *Francine Prince's New Gourmet Recipes for Dieters.*

# SOUPS

## THICK 'N SATISFYING BEEF-OKRA SOUP

It's as satisfying as it's simple to prepare. You're in for new taste thrills, too. The slight sweetness of okra and tomatoes, the pungency of garlic, the bite of curry highlight a perfect blendship of flavors. Marvelous preceded by a green salad and accompanied by my Best-Ever French Bread (page 152).

1 box (10 ounces) frozen okra
1 tablespoon white vinegar
1½ teaspoons each corn oil and Italian olive oil, combined
1 medium onion, minced
1 medium leek, white part plus 1 inch green part, well washed and minced
3 large cloves garlic, minced
½ pound lean top round of beef, cut into ½-inch cubes
1 tablespoon wine vinegar
1 cup apple juice (no sugar added)
2 cups water
1 teaspoon dried rosemary leaves, crushed
½ teaspoon dried thyme leaves, crushed
1½ teaspoons curry powder (no salt or pepper added)
3 tablespoons barley
Bouquet garni (2 sprigs fresh parsley, 1 bay leaf, tied together with white thread)

1. Bring a saucepan of water to rolling boil. Add white vinegar and okra. Boil for 2 minutes. Pour into strainer and then rinse under cold running water. Drain. Set aside.

2. Heat combined oils in nonstick skillet until hot. Add onion, leek, and garlic. Sauté over medium-high heat until lightly browned, stirring often. Add meat, combining with browned mixture, and sauté for 5 minutes, stirring every minute. Add wine vinegar. Sauté for 1 minute. Pour contents of skillet into kettle or stainless-steel pot.

3. Add balance of ingredients. Bring to simmering point. Reduce heat. Cover and simmer for 1½ hours, stirring every half hour. Turn off heat. Let stand, covered, for 20 minutes. Remove bouquet garni, reheat if necessary, and serve.

YIELD: Serves 4 as a main course, 6 as a first course

## UNTRADITIONAL GAZPACHO

Start with blanched, crispy green broccoli, crunchy cucumbers, and ripe fresh tomatoes. Then combine the slightly sweet and tart tastes of apple juice and vinegar, and point up the natural flavors of the ingredients with herbs and spices. The result is an *un*traditional gazpacho that searchers for new soup sensations will applaud.

1 cup broccoli flowerets

3 large cloves garlic, peeled, each clove cut in half

2 shallots, peeled, each shallot cut in half

1 crisp scallion, trimmed, cut into 6 pieces

2 large Kirby cucumbers, peeled and sliced

¼ cup fresh basil leaves, washed and dried

2 ripe tomatoes, skinned and coarsely chopped

⅛ teaspoon ground red (cayenne) pepper

½ teaspoon paprika

½ teaspoon curry powder (no salt or pepper added)

2 tablespoons wine vinegar

1 tablespoon each corn oil and Italian olive oil

½ teaspoon Worcestershire sauce (optional)

⅓ cup Miracle Chicken Stock (page 168)

¼ cup apple juice (no sugar added)

1 tablespoon each minced fresh parsley and dill

1. Drop broccoli flowerets into pot of rapidly boiling water and cook for 2 minutes. Pour into colander and drain. Place colander under cold running water and rinse broccoli until cooled.

2. Fit food processor with steel blade. Add broccoli and balance of ingredients to workbowl. Process on/off 6 times. Remove cover. Stir ingredients. Re-cover and process on/off several times until vegetables are finely chopped but not puréed. (You may have to remove cover again to check consistency.)

3. Serve chilled.

YIELD: Serves 4

SERVING SUGGESTION: Best-Ever French Bread (page 152) or Beginner's Loaf (page 150) make fine accompaniments to this soup.

## MUSHROOM-PEA SOUP

Meaty-tasting dried mushrooms, combined with split peas and flavored with spices and herbs, produce an exceptional, thick, deep-brown soup that not only satisfies vegetarians but meat lovers, too. A cinch to make!

½ ounce imported dried mushrooms, preferably the dark variety
⅓ cup water
1 tablespoon corn oil
3 large cloves garlic, minced
¾ cup thinly sliced leek (include white part and 1 inch of green part, well washed)
1 teaspoon peeled and minced fresh ginger
⅓ cup peeled and diced yellow turnip
1 tablespoon wine vinegar
½ cup dried split peas, well washed and drained
2 tablespoons barley, well washed and drained
2 cups each Miracle Chicken Stock (page 168) and water
⅓ cup apple juice (no sugar added)
2 teaspoons chili con carne seasoning (no salt or pepper added)
⅛ teaspoon ground red (cayenne) pepper
½ teaspoon ground marjoram
¼ teaspoon dried thyme leaves, crushed
Bouquet garni (3 sprigs parsley, 1 bay leaf, tied together with white thread)

1. Break mushrooms into small pieces. Place in cup. Add ⅓ cup water and let soak for 30 minutes.

2. Heat oil in stainless-steel pot or waterless cooker until hot. Add garlic, leek, and ginger and sauté over medium heat until wilted but not brown, stirring constantly. Add turnip. Stir. Add vinegar and cook for 1 minute.

3. Add mushrooms, mushroom liquid, and balance of ingredients. Bring to simmering point. Cover and simmer gently for 1¼ hours, stirring from time to time. Let stand, covered, for 30 minutes. Discard bouquet garni. Reheat if necessary, and serve.

YIELD: Serves 4

## LENTIL-PEA SOUP

Here's an exciting main course to replace a chicken with a vegetable dish. It's not really a soup, and it's not really a stew, but a lovely in-between with all the appeals of both. We love it on those first crisp evenings when autumn passes into winter.

¼ cup each dried lentils and split peas, washed and drained
1 small chicken breast with bone (¾ pound), plus 2 necks or wings, well trimmed and skinned
1½ tablespoons corn oil
3 large cloves garlic, minced
1 medium onion, minced
3 large fresh mushrooms, washed, trimmed, and coarsely chopped
1 small carrot, peeled and diced
½ cup diced white turnip
1 tablespoon tarragon or wine vinegar
¼ cup dry vermouth
4 cups water
½ teaspoon each dried thyme, sage, and rosemary leaves, crushed
1 tablespoon tomato paste (no salt added)
8 dashes ground red (cayenne) pepper
Bouquet garni (2 sprigs each fresh dill and parsley, 1 small bay leaf, tied together with white thread)

1. Soak lentils in water to cover overnight. Drain if necessary. Wash peas. Set lentils and peas aside.

2. Place chicken breast and necks or wings in kettle or stainless-steel pot with water to cover. Bring to boil. Boil for 2 minutes. Pour contents of kettle into colander. Wash under cold running water. Transfer to dish and set aside. Wash out kettle.

3. Heat oil in kettle until hot. Add garlic, onion, and mushrooms. Sauté until wilted but not brown, stirring often (about 3 minutes). Add carrot and turnip. Sauté for one minute. And vinegar and vermouth. Cook for 1 minute more. Return chicken pieces to kettle.

4. Add lentils, peas, and balance of ingredients. Bring to boil. Reduce heat to simmering. Cover and simmer for 1½ hours. Remove from heat and let stand for 15 minutes. Discard bouquet garni.

5. Remove chicken from bones. Cut into bite-size pieces. Return to soup. Stir to distribute evenly. Reheat if necessary, and serve.

YIELD: Serves 4

## TWO-WAY ZUCCHINI SOUP

Why is zucchini so popular? It's adaptable to many recipes, its calorie count is spectacularly low, and you can cook it in virtually no time at all. Available all year round, it's plentiful in summer, when it's much easier on your budget. This zucchini soup can be prepared two ways—as a liquid rich with chunky vegetables or as a smooth-as-velvet purée.

2 teaspoons corn oil
3 large cloves garlic, minced
1 each medium onion, minced, and leek, white part only, well washed and minced
3 medium zucchini (1¼ pounds), peeled and diced into ½-inch chunks
2 large ripe tomatoes (1½ pounds), cored, skinned, and coarsely chopped
2 tablespoons grated carrot
1½ cups Miracle Chicken Stock (page 168)
½ cup apple juice (no sugar added)
¼ cup dry vermouth
1 tablespoon fresh lemon juice
1 teaspoon each rosemary leaves, crushed, and curry powder (no salt or pepper added)
½ teaspoon cuminseed, crushed
2 dashes ground red (cayenne) pepper (optional)
1 tablespoon minced fresh parsley or dill

1. Heat oil in large stainless-steel pot or waterless cooker. Add garlic, onion, and leek. Sauté until just wilted, stirring with wooden spoon. Add zucchini and sauté for 1 minute.

2. Add balance of ingredients (except parsley or dill). Bring to simmering point. Partially cover and simmer for 15 minutes, stirring twice. Remove from heat. Let stand, partially covered, for 15 minutes.

3. Serve hot sprinkled with parsley or dill.

YIELD: About 5 cups; serves 6

VARIATION: Complete recipe through step 2. Then pour solids into blender and purée until smooth. (You may have to purée ingredients in 2 batches, depending upon the size of your blender.) Pour purée into bowl. Add liquid soup and stir with purée to blend. Pour into jar and chill. Sprinkle with parsley or dill and serve.

YIELD: About 4 cups; serves 6

NOTE: Many people prefer not to peel zucchini. If you can find the thin-skinned variety, scrub skin well and proceed with recipe.

# FIVE SALAD DRESSINGS, FOUR MARINADES, TWO TOPPINGS, A SAUCE, AND A STOCK

## FIVE SALAD DRESSINGS

Why settle for "diet" dressings when you can have the real thing with as little, or less, calories? Here are five delicious dressings, one of which—a mayonnaise-type dressing—doubles as a spread. They're so easy to make, and so delicious, you'll give up that bottled stuff forever. Find your favorite by trying them all. But take warning: you may end up, as my family did, with five favorites.

### ALL-PURPOSE SALAD DRESSING

¼ cup corn oil
1 tablespoon each fresh lemon juice and apple cider vinegar
½ cup cold Miracle Chicken Stock (page 168)
½ teaspoon dried mustard
1 tablespoon minced dried onion
2 tablespoons tomato juice (no salt added)
½ teaspoon garlic powder
6 dashes ground red (cayenne) pepper
1 teaspoon minced fresh tarragon or ½ teaspoon dried tarragon leaves, crushed
1 tablespoon minced fresh parsley

1. Place all ingredients in jar, shaking well to blend. Let stand for at least 1 hour before serving. Shake again before serving.

YIELD: About 1 cup

NOTE: This dressing will keep fresh for 2 to 3 days in tightly closed jar in refrigerator.

### LOW-CALORIE TOMATO SALAD DRESSING

¼ cup each evaporated skim milk and tomato juice (no salt added)
3 tablespoons dry-curd cottage cheese (no salt added)
1 scallion, minced
¼ teaspoon each dried sweet basil leaves, crushed, and curry powder (no salt or pepper added)
1 tablespoon fresh lemon juice
1 teaspoon wine vinegar
3 tablespoons plain low-fat yogurt
1 tablespoon minced fresh parsley or dill

Place all ingredients in small bowl. Beat with wire whisk until blended. Or purée all ingredients in electric blender until smooth.

YIELD: 1 cup

VARIATIONS:
1. Add 1 tablespoon corn oil to recipe. Place all ingredients in electric blender and blend until smooth.
2. One tablespoon minced shallot or onion may be substituted for scallion.

NOTE: This dressing will keep fresh for 1 to 2 days in tightly closed jar in refrigerator.

## LIME SALAD DRESSING

⅓ cup corn oil
3 tablespoons fresh lime juice
2 tablespoons water or Miracle
    Chicken Stock (page 168)
1 large shallot, minced
2 cloves garlic, minced
6 dashes ground red (cayenne) pepper
½ teaspoon each dried marjoram and
    rosemary leaves, crushed

## FRUIT SALAD DRESSING

1 tablespoon fresh lemon juice
1 teaspoon apple cider vinegar
¼ cup each orange and pineapple juice
    (no sugar added)
2 tablespoons corn oil
¼ teaspoon each cuminseed, crushed,
    and ground cinnamon
2 dashes ground red (cayenne) pepper
¼ cup loosely packed minced fresh
    basil

Combine all ingredients in jar and shake well. Let stand for 30 minutes before serving. Shake again before serving.

YIELD: About ⅔ cup

NOTE: This dressing will keep fresh for 2 to 3 days in tightly closed jar in refrigerator.

Combine all ingredients except basil in jar. Shake to blend. Stir in minced basil. Serve immediately.

YIELD: About ½ cup; enough to serve 4

VARIATIONS:

1. Add ¼ cup sliced ripe banana to recipe. Combine first 6 listed ingredients in electric blender with banana. Purée until smooth. Stir in minced basil and serve over salad that includes banana.

2. Add ¼ teaspoon curry powder (no salt or pepper added) to recipe.

3. One tablespoon minced fresh tarragon, rosemary, or dill may be substituted for fresh basil.

NOTE: This basic dressing will keep fresh for up to 2 to 3 days in tightly closed jar in refrigerator. Variation 1 tastes best if used first day.

## ALMOST MAYONNAISE

2 tablespoons each evaporated skim milk, tomato juice (no salt added), and dry-curd cottage cheese
1 tablespoon minced shallot
½ teaspoon each curry powder (no salt or pepper added), and dried tarragon leaves, crushed
2 teaspoons fresh lemon juice
½ teaspoon wine vinegar
1 tablespoon minced fresh parsley
½ teaspoon prepared Dijon mustard (no salt added)
1 egg yolk
6 dashes ground red (cayenne) pepper
1 tablespoon Italian olive oil
¼ cup corn oil

1. Place first 6 listed ingredients in small bowl. Beat with wire whisk until smooth. Set aside.

2. Fit food processor with steel blade. To workbowl add mustard, egg yolk, ground red pepper, and olive oil. Process for 60 seconds. Then dribble corn oil through feed tube with machine on. (Mixture will be very thick.)

3. With machine on, slowly pour whisked mixture through feed tube until well puréed. Mixture will be a perfect consistency as a salad dressing. For a thicker consistency to use as a spread, pour into jar and refrigerate until well chilled.

YIELD: ⅔ cup

NOTE: Mayonnaise may be successfully prepared with wire whisk alone. Here's how: Follow step 1. In another bowl add mustard, egg yolk, ground red pepper, and 1 tablespoon Italian olive oil. Beat with wire whisk until well blended. Then dribble corn oil into bowl while beating with whisk until all oil is absorbed. (Mixture will be thick.) Slowly add mixture from step 1, beating well until absorbed.

## FOUR MARINADES

These delectable mixtures of vinegars, juices, herbs, and spices transform plain roasts, chops, or poultry into exquisite flavor delights. They're quick and simple to prepare, and they take a good deal of the guesswork out of cooking. For basic instructions on how to use any of these marinades on meat or poultry, see pages 117 and 134 respectively.

### VERSATILE MARINADE

2 tablespoons partially thawed orange juice concentrate (no sugar added)
¼ cup apple juice (no sugar added)
2 tablespoons apple cider vinegar
2 tablespoons corn oil
½ teaspoon each ground ginger and marjoram
¼ teaspoon ground sage
⅛ teaspoon ground red (cayenne) pepper
½ teaspoon Worcestershire sauce
3 large cloves garlic, minced
1 tablespoon combined minced fresh parsley and dill

Combine all ingredients in jar. Shake well to blend.

YIELD: About ¾ cup; enough to marinate a 3½-pound chicken or roast

### HERB MARINADE I

¼ cup apple juice (no sugar added)
3 tablespoons apple cider vinegar
2 tablespoons dry vermouth
2 tablespoons corn oil
3 cloves garlic, minced
2 large shallots, minced
½-inch slice fresh ginger, peeled and shredded
8 dashes ground red (cayenne) pepper
1 teaspoon dry mustard
1 teaspoon dried rosemary leaves, crushed
1 tablespoon minced fresh parsley

Combine all ingredients in jar. Shake well to blend.

YIELD: About ¾ cup; enough to marinate up to a 3½-pound chicken or roast

NOTE: This marinade can also be used with fish.

## HERB MARINADE II

¼ cup wine vinegar
3 tablespoons apple cider vinegar
1 teaspoon each dried savory leaves and sage leaves, crushed
⅛ teaspoon ground red (cayenne) pepper
2 tablespoons corn oil
2 tablespoons partially thawed apple juice concentrate (no sugar added)
1 teaspoon chili con carne seasoning (no salt or pepper added)
3 large shallots, minced
2 large cloves garlic, minced

Combine all ingredients in jar. Shake well to blend.

YIELD: About ¾ cup; enough to marinate up to a 3½-pound chicken or roast.

NOTE: This marinade can also be used with fish.

## MIDDLE-EAST MARINADE

3 cloves garlic, minced
1 tablespoon wine vinegar
1 tablespoon corn oil
¼ cup Miracle Chicken Stock (page 168)
2 tablespoons dry vermouth
2 tablespoons apple juice (no sugar added)
1 tablespoon minced fresh parsley
1 teaspoon dried rosemary leaves, crushed
½ teaspoon cuminseed, crushed
1 teaspoon curry powder (no salt or pepper added)
8 dashes ground red (cayenne) pepper

Combine all ingredients in jar. Shake well to blend.

YIELD: About ½ cup; enough to marinate up to a 3½-pound chicken or roast

# TWO TOPPINGS

One is for desserts; the other, for cold fish, chicken, and salads. Both are so luxuriously creamy you would think they're forbidden foods. Dieting was never like this!

## WHIPPED CREAMY TOPPING

⅓ cup evaporated skim milk
1 teaspoon grated orange rind, preferably from navel orange
¼ teaspoon ground cinnamon

1. Pour milk into large mixing bowl. Place bowl and whipping untensils in freezer. Chill until fine crystals begin to form around edges. Whip until stiff (mixture will whip up as stiffly as whole cream if milk and utensils are sufficiently cold.)

2. Stir in orange rind and ground cinnamon and serve.

YIELD: Serves 6

VARIATIONS: Allspice, nutmeg, and pure vanilla extract may be substituted for orange rind and cinnamon. Or basic recipe may be used with the addition of your choice of spices to taste. Always beat the cold milk first before adding balance of ingredients.

## RICH-TASTING TOMATO TOPPING

¼ cup evaporated skim milk
2 medium tomatoes
2 large shallots, minced
8 dashes ground red (cayenne) pepper
½ teaspoon curry powder (no salt or pepper added)
¼ cup minced fresh basil (see note below)

1. Pour milk into large mixing bowl. Follow directions for Whipped Creamy Topping (above).
2. Choose ripe tomatoes. Drop into pot of boiling water. Let boil for 1 minute. Drain and cool. Peel and core, taking care not to lose tomato juices. Coarsely chop. Place in electric blender or processor.

3. Add shallots and spices to blender. Blend on high speed until smooth. Pour into large bowl. Stir in minced basil. Then fold in whipped milk. (Do not overfold.)
4. Serve over broiled or poached fish (hot or cold), cold chicken or turkey, and salads.

YIELD: Serves 6

NOTE: Fresh herbs taste best. If fresh basil isn't available, you can successfully substitute 2 tablespoons minced fresh tarragon, rosemary, or 1 tablespoon each minced fresh parsley and dill.

# A SAUCE . . .

## CREAMY GREEN SAUCE

Here's a simple and quick-to-make dieter's delight that doubles as a dip. It's sheer magic on poached fish and vegetables, and transforms an ordinary salad into an extraordinary one. It's also a feast for the eye. Try the variations, too. Then come up with your own. They could surpass mine.

⅔ cup dry-curd cottage cheese (no salt added)
¼ cup buttermilk (no salt added)
1 tablespoon evaporated skim milk
6 dashes ground red (cayenne) pepper
1 tablespoon combined minced fresh parsley and mint
1 medium scallion (use the green part too), coarsely chopped

1. Combine all ingredients in electric blender or processor and blend on high speed until well puréed. Sauce will turn a delicate green and should be very smooth.
2. Pour into jar and refrigerate until ready to use.

YIELD: ⅔ cup

VARIATIONS:

1. Combine first 4 ingredients in electric blender. Add 1 tablespoon grated onion, ½ teaspoon curry powder (no salt or pepper added), and 2 teaspoons minced fresh parsley. Blend.

2. Add 1 teaspoon tomato paste (no salt added) to basic recipe. Blend.

3. Combine first 4 ingredients in electric blender. Add 1 tablespoon combined minced fresh dill and parsley, 1 teaspoon grated carrot, and ⅛ teaspoon anise or fennel seeds, crushed. Blend.

NOTE: Sauce tastes best freshly made, but will keep for 1 day in tightly closed jar in refrigerator.

# ... AND A STOCK

## MIRACLE CHICKEN STOCK

Stock, a highly concentrated clear broth, is to my way of thinking the simplest and most delicious way to enrich many dishes. Just try it on one of my dishes calling for stock—say, Mushroom-Pea Soup (page 158)—and you'll understand what a boon it is, particularly when you cook without salt. It's simple to make (it simmers away while you're free as a bird), and it requires less ingredients than most recipes. I stock up on stock (see note). Why can't you?

3½ pounds chicken giblets (excluding liver), backs, and wings, or 1 broiling chicken and giblets (3½ pounds), skinned and quartered
4 large cloves garlic, minced
1 medium leek, white part plus 2 inches green part, well washed and diced
1 medium onion, peeled and quartered
½-inch slice fresh ginger, peeled and shredded
1 medium carrot, peeled and sliced
1 medium parsnip, peeled and diced
1 large white turnip, peeled and diced
1 rib celery, diced
4 large fresh mushrooms, well washed and trimmed
½ cup dry vermouth
7 cups water
Bouquet garni (3 sprigs parsley, 1 bay leaf, tied together with white thread)

1. Place giblets or chicken in large stainless-steel pot or waterless cooker. Cover with water. Bring to rolling boil. Boil for 1 minute. Place colander in sink. Pour contents of pot into colander and drain. Rinse under cold running water to remove all scum from chicken. Wash out pot. Return contents of colander to pot.

2. Add balance of ingredients to pot. Bring to rolling boil. Turn heat down to slow boil. Partially cover and simmer gently for 2½ hours, removing any additional scum that rises to top after first 10 minutes of cooking. Let stock cool in pot.

3. With slotted spoon, remove chicken from broth. (Enjoy chicken as is, or try my delicious New Chicken Salad, page 185.) Place fine-meshed strainer or chinois over bowl. Pour balance of ingredients into strainer, pressing broth out of solids. Discard solids.

4. Transfer stock to freezeproof containers. Refrigerate some broth for use within a few days and freeze the balance.

YIELD: About 5 cups

VARIATION: For a pleasant and subtle flavor, change water measurement to 6 cups and add 1 cup apple juice (no sugar added).

NOTE: Prepare stock just once a month. Then freeze in 1-cup containers as well as in ice-cube trays. That gives you instantly available measured amounts.

# HORS D'OEUVRES

You'll find these colorfully presented fragments of deliciousness to be perfect gastronomic preludes to any of my meals. Enjoy them often with an easy mind. They contribute nary an ounce to your next day's weigh-in.

## WONDER HORS D'OEUVRE

1 bunch crisp arrugula, each leaf well washed and dried

1 medium ripe mango, peeled and cut into ½-inch thick slices

Place each slice of mango in center of each arrugula leaf. Fold each side of leaf over lengthwise. Secure with cocktail picks. Serve well chilled.

YIELD: About 20 hors d'oeuvres

VARIATION: Any ripe melon in season—such as honeydew, cantaloupe, or casaba—may be substituted for mango. The emphasis is on *ripe*.

## COLORFUL SHRIMP CANAPÉS

¼ pound fresh medium shrimp, unshelled
   Bouquet garni (2 sprigs fresh dill, 1 bay leaf, tied together with white thread)
1 tablespoon fresh lime juice
2 shallots, minced
1 small carrot, peeled and grated
2 tablespoons each minced celery and sweet red pepper
1 tablespoon each minced fresh dill and parsley
3 tablespoons plain low-fat yogurt
6 dashes each paprika and ground red (cayenne) pepper
1 teaspoon tomato paste (no salt added)
½ teaspoon dried tarragon leaves, crushed
3 slices Beginner's Loaf (page 150) or whole-wheat bread

1. Bring saucepan of water to rolling boil. Add shrimp and bouquet garni. Reduce heat to medium boil and cook shrimp for 5 minutes. Pour into colander and drain. Then place under cold running water until cooled. Shell and devein. Dry on paper toweling and coarsely chop. Place shrimp in bowl. Sprinkle with lime juice and toss.

2. Add shallots, carrot, celery, sweet red pepper, dill, and parsley. Toss to blend.

3. Combine and blend yogurt with paprika, ground red pepper, tomato paste and tarragon. Pour over shrimp mixture and stir until shrimp are well coated.

4. Spread on bread slices, pressing mixture firmly into bread. Cut each slice into quarters and serve.

YIELD: 12 canapes

VARIATION: To serve as a salad for two, omit bread and pile shrimp mixture into crisp lettuce cups. Surround with radish flowers, sliced tomatoes, and crisp watercress.

## TASTY TUNA HORS D'OEUVRES

1 can (6½ ounces) tuna, packed in water (no salt added)
1 tablespoon fresh lemon juice
2 tablespoons dry-curd cottage cheese (no salt added)
2 tablespoons each minced scallion, sweet red pepper, and celery
1 teaspoon curry powder (no salt or pepper added)
1 tablespoon minced fresh tarragon or 1½ teaspoons dried tarragon leaves, crushed
1 tablespoon minced fresh parsley
8 dashes ground red (cayenne) pepper
About ¼ cup All-Purpose Salad Dressing (page 161)
6 slices firm-textured bread, such as Beginner's Loaf (page 150)

1. Drain water from can. Turn tuna into bowl, sprinkle with lemon juice, and mash. Mash cheese into mixture.
2. Stir in balance of ingredients, except salad dressing and bread. Then add only enough salad dressing to moisten.
3. Spread tuna mixture on bread slices. Cut each slice into 3 triangles.

YIELD: 18 hors d'oeuvres

VARIATION: Cut tops from 4 medium tomatoes. Remove pulp in one piece. Fill with tuna mixture. Replace pulp on top of mixture. Surround with crisp watercress, cucumbers, and radish flowers.

## THREE-WAY EGGPLANT CAVIAR

Serve as an hors d'oeuvre, a dip, or a relish.

1 eggplant (1 pound)
2 large ripe tomatoes (¾ pound)
3 large cloves garlic, minced
2 large shallots, minced
1 medium onion, minced
1 tablespoon each minced fresh parsley and dill
1 tablespoon wine vinegar
2 tablespoons fresh lemon juice
8 dashes ground red (cayenne) pepper
½ teaspoon curry powder (no salt or pepper added)
2 teaspoons tomato paste (no salt added)
1 teaspoon Worcestershire sauce

1. Prick eggplant with sharp-pronged fork. Place on a sheet of aluminum foil and bake in preheated 400°F oven for 45 minutes. (Eggplant will turn black and skin will easily peel off.) Let cool. Dice.

2. Drop tomatoes into boiling water for 1 minute. Core and peel. Let cool. Dice.

3. Place diced eggplant and tomatoes in bowl. Add balance of ingredients, one at a time, stirring gently after each addition. (Do not mash.) Serve chilled.

YIELD: 3 cups

NOTES:

1. I recommend preparing this recipe a day ahead for greatest flavor enjoyment.

2. If you have a food processor, cut baked eggplant and tomatoes into large chunks. Add to workbowl. Turn processor on/off 3 times. Transfer mixture to another bowl. Add garlic, shallots, large chunks of onion, and parsley and dill flowerets to work bowl. Process on/off 3 times. Add to eggplant mixture. Continue with balance of recipe.

## PICKLED BRUSSELS SPROUTS

¾ pound small fresh Brussels sprouts, trimmed, cooked 15 minutes in rapidly boiling water, and cooled
2 teaspoons pickling spices
⅓ cup combined apple cider vinegar and wine vinegar
1 tablespoon fresh lime juice
2 tablespoons apple juice (no sugar added)
1 large shallot, minced
1 large clove garlic, minced
6 dashes ground red (cayenne) pepper
1 tablespoon combined minced fresh parsley and dill
¼ teaspoon dried thyme leaves, crushed

1. Place cooled Brussels sprouts in small bowl.

2. Combine balance of ingredients in saucepan. Bring to simmering point. Cover and simmer gently for 5 minutes. Strain into bowl with Brussels sprouts. Stir and spoon liquid over sprouts. Let stand at room temperature for 30 minutes, stirring often.

3. Transfer to jar. Cover tightly and refrigerate overnight, turning jar upside down from time to time. Serve cold, pierced with colorful cocktail picks.

YIELD: About 20 sprouts; serves 4

# BREAKFAST DISHES

*Yes,* pancakes, French toast, muffins, and omelets! There's no reason why a dieter can't expand the joys of the most important meal of the day. Here are five delectable alternates to shredded wheat and whole-wheat toast.

## HEARTY CREAM OF WHEAT

2 cups water
¼ cup apple juice (no sugar added)
⅓ cup Cream of Wheat cereal
1 tablespoon unprocessed bran
½ teaspoon ground coriander
¼ teaspoon ground cinnamon
2 tablespoons toasted wheat germ (no sugar added)

1. Combine water and apple juice in saucepan. Bring to boil. Sprinkle with Cream of Wheat, bran, and spices, stirring constantly. Reduce heat and cook for 8 minutes, stirring occasionally.

2. Pour into serving dish. Sprinkle with wheat germ and serve.

YIELD: Serves 2

VARIATION: Add 2 tablespoons evaporated skim milk to saucepan at the completion of step 1, stirring to blend.

NOTE: For added fiber in all of your cooked breakfast cereals, add 1 to 2 tablespoons unprocessed bran during cooking process, or stir in just before serving.

## COTTAGE CHEESE PANCAKE

2 eggs (use 1 yolk and 2 whites)
¼ cup dry-curd cottage cheese (no salt added)
¼ cup evaporated skim milk
2 tablespoons each nonfat liquid milk and fresh orange juice
¼ cup plus 1 tablespoon unbleached flour
1 teaspoon low-sodium baking powder
⅛ teaspoon freshly grated nutmeg
½ teaspoon ground cinnamon
½ teaspoon grated orange rind, preferably from navel orange
1 tablespoon sweet (unsalted) 100 percent corn oil margarine, for pan
1 tablespoon fresh lemon juice

1. Combine eggs, cottage cheese, milks, and orange juice in electric blender. Sift ¼ cup flour, baking powder, and spices into blender. Blend on medium speed until smooth (about 10 seconds). Stir in balance of flour and orange rind.

2. Heat 10-inch well-seasoned iron skillet (see note 2 below) until hot. Add margarine and heat until melted, tilting skillet from side to side so entire surface is moistened. Pour batter into hot skillet. Cook over medium-high heat for 30 seconds. Place in preheated 425°F oven and bake for 15 to 18 minutes. Mixture will puff up and turn a golden brown on top. Bottom of pancake should be browned.

3. Slide pancake onto warmed serving plate. Sprinkle with lemon juice and serve immediately.

YIELD: Serves 4

VARIATION: Add 1 tablespoon unprocessed bran for added fiber. You'll never know it's there!

NOTES:

1. Makes a fine lunch dish, too.

2. For directions on how to prepare a well-seasoned iron skillet, see note for Savory Sautéed Chicken on page 130.

## BLUEBERRY MUFFINS I

1 egg
3 tablespoons corn oil
½ teaspoon grated lemon rind
¾ cup nonfat liquid milk
2 tablespoons evaporated skim milk
2 tablespoons honey
1½ cups unbleached flour
4 teaspoons low-sodium baking powder (available in health food stores)
½ teaspoon ground cinnamon
2 tablespoons toasted wheat germ (no sugar added)
1 tablespoon date sugar (date powder; available in health food stores)
1 cup fresh blueberries, picked over, washed, and patted dry with paper toweling
½ teaspoon sweet (unsalted) 100 percent corn oil margarine, for muffin pans

1. In bowl, combine egg, oil, and lemon rind. Beat with wooden spoon until blended. Stir in milks and honey.

2. Sift flour, baking powder, and cinnamon into egg mixture. Stir in wheat germ and date sugar. Blend well.

3. Fold in blueberries.

4. Half-fill margarine-greased 3-inch muffin pans with batter. Bake in preheated 400°F oven for 20 to 22 minutes, until browned. (A well-browned, crunchy muffin will be more satisfying than a soft one.)

5. Remove pan from oven. Place on rack and let cool for 5 minutes. Loosen muffins with blunt knife. Invert pan. Turn muffins right side up. Let cool on rack. Serve slightly warm.

YIELD: 12 muffins

NOTE: Great for dessert at any meal.

## BLUEBERRY MUFFINS II

1 egg
3 tablespoons corn oil
3 tablespoons honey
½ teaspoon grated orange rind, preferably from navel orange
1¼ cups unbleached flour
⅓ cup whole-wheat flour
4 teaspoons low-sodium baking powder (available in health food stores)
½ cup evaporated skim milk
⅓ cup plain low-fat yogurt
½ teaspoon pure vanilla extract
1 cup fresh blueberries, picked over, washed, and patted dry with paper toweling
½ teaspoon sweet (unsalted) 100 percent corn oil margarine, for muffin pans

1. Combine egg, oil, honey, and orange rind in bowl. Beat with wooden spoon until blended.

2. Sift flours and baking powder into another bowl. Combine milk and yogurt in cup, stirring to blend. Add sifted ingredients alternately with milk mixture to egg mixture (step 1), a little at a time, stirring only until blended. (Do not beat.) Stir in vanilla.

3. Fold in blueberries.

4. Half-fill margarine-greased 3-inch muffin pans with batter. Bake in preheated 400°F oven for 20 to 22 minutes, until browned.

5. Remove pan from oven. Place on rack and let cool for 5 minutes. Loosen muffins with blunt knife. Invert pan. Turn muffins right side up. Let cool on rack. Serve slightly warm.

YIELD: 12 muffins

NOTE: Why not try these as a dessert for lunch or dinner?

## LIGHT-AS-A-FEATHER BRAN MUFFINS

2 tablespoons each corn oil and room-temperature sweet (unsalted) 100 percent corn oil margarine
2 tablespoons honey
2 eggs (use 1 yolk and 2 whites)
2 teaspoons grated orange rind, preferably from navel orange
1 tablespoon partially thawed orange juice concentrate (no sugar added)
½ cup buttermilk (no salt added)
1 cup unbleached flour
4½ teaspoons low-sodium baking powder (available in health food stores)
½ teaspoon ground cinnamon
¼ teaspoon ground allspice
1 cup unprocessed bran
⅓ cup raisins
½ teaspoon margarine for muffin pans

1. Combine 2 tablespoons each oil and margarine in mixing bowl. Beat with whisk until combined. Add honey, eggs, and orange rind. Whisk until smooth. Add orange juice concentrate and buttermilk. Whisk only until concentrate is dissolved.

2. Sift flour, baking powder, and spices into mixture. Whisk until smooth. With wooden spoon, stir in bran and raisins.

3. Fill margarine-greased 3-inch muffin cups two-thirds full with batter. Bake in preheated 400°F oven for 15 to 17 minutes, until muffins are delicately brown on top.

4. Place pan on rack and let cool for 5 minutes. With blunt knife, loosen around each muffin, then lift muffins out of pans. They'll come out easily. Serve warm.

YIELD: 9 large muffins

NOTES:

1. For smaller muffins, half-fill 12 margarine-greased muffin cups with batter. Bake for 13 to 15 minutes, or until delicately browned on top.

2. These will be mouth-watering desserts at your other meals as well.

## BANANA FRENCH TOAST

8 (1-inch thick) slices day-old Best-Ever French Bread (page 152), or commercial French or Italian bread
2 eggs (use 1 yolk and 2 whites)
½ medium banana, sliced
¼ cup evaporated skim milk
½ teaspoon each ground cinnamon and coriander
2 dashes ground red (cayenne) pepper
2 teaspoons corn oil

1. Place sliced bread in wide bowl.
2. Combine eggs, banana, skim milk, and spices in electric blender. Blend until smooth. Pour over bread, saturating slices well. Let soak for 10 minutes, spooning often with banana mixture. (Most of liquid should be absorbed.)
3. Heat 1 teaspoon corn oil in non-stick skillet until hot. Add bread slices, spooning any unabsorbed liquid over them. Sauté over medium-high heat until brown on both sides, adding balance of oil just before turning.
4. Serve immediately, sprinkled with ground cinnamon or spooned with your favorite honey.

NOTE: Any reason why you can't have French toast for lunch?

## WESTERN-STYLE OMELET

### *For the filling:*

2 teaspoons corn oil
2 tablespoons each minced sweet green or red pepper and onion
2 large fresh mushrooms, washed, dried, trimmed, and coarsely chopped
2 dashes ground red (cayenne) pepper
½ teaspoon dried basil leaves, crushed, or 1 tablespoon minced fresh basil
1 teaspoon tomato paste (no salt added)
2 tablespoons evaporated skim milk

### *For the omelet:*

3 eggs (use ½ of one yolk and all of whites)
¼ teaspoon garlic powder
½ teaspoon curry powder (no salt or pepper added)
1 teaspoon each minced fresh parsley and dill, combined
4 dashes ground red (cayenne) pepper
1 tablespoon evaporated skim milk
½ teaspoon corn oil, for pan

1. Prepare filling first. Heat oil in nonstick skillet until hot. Sauté sweet pepper, onion, and mushrooms over medium-high heat, stirring constantly, until lightly browned. Sprinkle with ground red pepper and basil. Stir.

2. Combine tomato paste with milk. Reduce heat under skillet. Add tomato paste mixture. Cook briefly until vegetables are heated through. Transfer to small bowl. Cover to keep warm. Wipe out skillet.

3. To prepare omelet, combine first 6 ingredients in small bowl. Beat with wire whisk until well blended.

4. Brush nonstick skillet lightly with oil. Heat until hot but not smoking. Pour egg mixture into pan, tilting pan from side to side so mixture covers surface evenly. Cook until lightly browned on one side only (the center should remain moist). Slide onto dish. Place filling on one half of circle. Flip other half of circle over filling. Cut omelet in half and serve immediately on warmed plate.

YIELD: Serves 2

VARIATION: Substitute ½ teaspoon chili con carne seasoning (no salt or pepper added) for curry powder, and add ½ teaspoon wine vinegar at end of step 1.

NOTE: Makes a perfect lunch dish as well.

# SALADS

There are two kinds of salads. You eat one kind *before* your entrée; the other kind, *as* your entrée. In these ten salads you'll find exciting *new* varieties of both kinds.

Salads are a dieter's best friend; you can eat mounds of the *before*-your-entrée-kind without gaining an ounce. A chicory leaf has only three calories; an endive leaf, two; and a lettuce leaf, just one. All salads fill you up because they're packed with nature's appetite suppressant, fiber.

And one more reason for going steady with salads. They can be delicious. They *are* here.

## ARRUGULA SALAD

1 bunch arrugula, well washed and dried

2 ripe medium tomatoes, cored and cut into small wedges

2 Kirby cucumbers, scrubbed and sliced

4 scallions, sliced, or 1 medium sweet onion, thinly sliced

½ pound fresh mushrooms, washed, dried, trimmed, and sliced

2 tablespoons minced fresh parsley or 1 tablespoon each minced fresh parsley and dill

¼ teaspoon paprika
Lime Salad Dressing (page 162)

1. Prepare salad just before serving. Combine all ingredients except salad dressing in salad bowl. Toss gently.

2. Add only enough salad dressing to moisten (allow up to 2 tablespoons per serving). Toss to coat. Serve immediately.

YIELD: Serves 4

VARIATION: Serve salad with All-Purpose Salad Dressing (page 161), allowing 2 tablespoons per serving, or with Low-Calorie Tomato Salad Dressing (page 161), using as much dressing as you like.

## BASIL TOMATO SALAD

½ cup cooked brown rice, chilled
2 large ripe but firm tomatoes, cored, peeled, and coarsely chopped
2 medium Kirby cucumbers, peeled and cut into ½-inch cubes
2 whole scallions, cut diagonally into ½-inch pieces
1 large shallot, minced
¼ cup All-Purpose Salad Dressing (page 161)
⅛ teaspoon ground red (cayenne) pepper
½ teaspoon fennel seeds, well crushed
⅓ cup loosely packed minced fresh basil (see note)

1. Place first 5 ingredients in salad bowl. Toss.
2. Combine salad dressing, ground red pepper, and crushed seeds in jar, shaking to blend. Pour over salad. Toss to blend.
3. Gently fold in minced basil. Serve immediately.

YIELD: Serves 4

VARIATION: If you're lucky enough to find wild rice in your area and your budget allows you to splurge, substitute ¼ cup uncooked wild rice for cooked brown rice, following cooking directions on the package. Do not overcook. Chill. The results are chewy and delicious.

NOTE: Only fresh herbs will do here. If fresh basil isn't available, substitute 3 tablespoons minced fresh tarragon, rosemary, mint, or dill.

## CRUNCHY ROMAINE SALAD

1 small head romaine lettuce
2 medium red onions, peeled and thinly sliced
2 medium sweet red peppers, seeded and cut into ⅜-inch slivers
All-Purpose Salad Dressing (page 161)

1. Remove each leaf of romaine and wash under cold running water. Wipe dry with paper toweling (do not squeeze dry). Break leaves into bite-size pieces, discarding tough center stalk.

Drop into salad bowl. Add onions and peppers. Toss to combine.

2. Add only enough salad dressing to moisten salad, allowing up to 2 tablespoons per serving. Toss to coat.

YIELD: Serves 4

VARIATIONS: Serve salad with Lime Salad Dressing (page 162), allowing 2 tablespoons per serving, or with Low-Calorie Tomato Salad Dressing (page 161), using as much dressing as you like.

## LUNCHEON FRUIT SALAD

1 small bunch crisp watercress
1 small head romaine lettuce
1 small carrot, peeled and shredded
1 cup shredded red cabbage
2 navel oranges, peeled and cut into
  ½-inch chunks
¼ cup raisins (optional)
½ cup Fruit Salad Dressing (page 162).

1. Wash watercress and romaine under cold running water. Dry thoroughly with paper toweling. Break off and discard tough stems from watercress. Cut away thick outer leaves and center sections from romaine. Tear romaine into 1-inch pieces. Place watercress and romaine in salad bowl.

2. If you have a food processor, fit with shredding blade and shred carrot and cabbage. If you don't have a processor, grate carrot and cabbage through large holes of hand grater. (Cabbage may also be thinly sliced.) Combine with watercress and romaine.

3. Add oranges, raisins, and dressing. Toss gently, and serve.

YIELD: Serves 4

SUBSTITUTIONS: Any of the following fresh fruits in the quantities designated may be substituted for oranges:

- 3 medium nectarines or peaches
- 1 cup small melon balls
- 2 ripe bananas, sliced
- 1 ripe medium mango, peeled and sliced
- 2 large crisp sweet apples, cored and diced
- 1 cup sweet fresh Hawaiian pineapple, diced
- 1 cup canned pineapple tidbits in their own juice

## NEW CHICKEN SALAD

3 cups cooked skinned chicken, cut into ½-inch cubes, chilled
1 tablespoon fresh lemon juice
1 tablespoon wine vinegar
1 medium sweet red pepper, seeded and cut into ¼-inch slivers
⅓ cup shredded carrot
1 medium onion, thinly sliced
1 small rib celery, diced
1 large navel orange, peeled, sectioned, and cut into 1-inch chunks
½ cup well-scrubbed, sliced (¼-inch thick) zucchini
2 tablespoons each minced fresh dill and parsley
½ teaspoon cuminseed, well crushed
1 teaspoon curry powder (no salt or pepper added)
6 tablespoons All-Purpose Salad Dressing (page 161)
Crisp lettuce leaves and watercress sprigs

1. Place chicken in large bowl. Sprinkle with lemon juice and vinegar. Toss gently.

2. Add sweet red pepper, carrot, onion, celery, orange, zucchini, and minced herbs. Toss briefly.

3. Combine cuminseed and curry powder with salad dressing in cup, beating with fork to blend. Pour over salad. Stir until vegetables, fruit, and chicken are moistened. Let stand for 30 minutes before serving, stirring once.

4. Arrange on lettuce leaves, garnished with crisp watercress sprigs.

## OLD-FASHIONED COLE SLAW

2½ cups shredded tender green cabbage
2 medium carrots, peeled and shredded
1 medium sweet green pepper, shredded
2 tablespoons fresh lemon juice
1 tablespoon each apple cider vinegar and wine vinegar
2 tablespoons apple juice (no sugar added)
3 tablespoons plain low-fat yogurt
1 tablespoon each minced fresh parsley and dill
6 dashes ground red (cayenne) pepper
3 tablespoons Almost Mayonnaise (page 163)

1. Place shredded cabbage, carrots, and green pepper in large bowl. Add lemon juice, vinegars, and apple juice. Toss.

2. Stir in yogurt and minced fresh herbs. Sprinkle with ground red pepper and blend. Add mayonnaise, stirring until all ingredients are evenly blended.

3. Turn into covered refrigerator container or jar and chill for several hours (or overnight) before serving, stirring from time to time.

YIELD: Serves 6

VARIATIONS:

1. Add 1 small onion, minced, in step 1.

2. Add ¼ cup raisins in step 2.

3. Sprinkle each portion with ½ teaspoon coarsely chopped walnuts or almonds.

4. Add 2 ounces trimmed and blanched fresh snow peas to recipe, cutting each snow pea into thirds.

## PERFECT 10 CUCUMBER SALAD

1 pound Kirby cucumbers, well scrubbed and thinly sliced

1 small onion, thinly sliced and separated into rings

1 medium sweet red pepper, seeded and cut into ⅛-inch slivers

¼ cup wine vinegar

⅛ teaspoon ground red (cayenne) pepper

2 tablespoons minced fresh dill

2 tablespoons apple juice (no sugar added)

1 tablespoon honey

½ teaspoon curry powder (no salt or pepper added)

⅓ cup plain low-fat yogurt

1. Place first 3 ingredients in bowl.

2. Combine and blend balance of ingredients, except yogurt, in small bowl. Pour over vegetables. Toss gently.

3. Add yogurt, stirring to blend. Let stand for 10 minutes before serving.

YIELD: Serves 4

NOTE: Salad tastes best if eaten within 1 hour.

## SNOW PEA AND BEANSPROUT SALAD

¼ pound fresh snow peas, washed, dried, stems and strings removed

1 cup mung bean sprouts, washed and drained on paper toweling

1 ripe tomato, cored, peeled, and cut into chunks

3 to 4 tablespoons Lime Salad Dressing (page 162)
Crisp romaine lettuce leaves

1 tablespoon unsalted coarsely chopped almonds

1. Blanch snow peas by dropping them into a saucepan of rapidly boiling water for 1 minute. Pour into colander and drain. Place colander under cold running water to stop cooking action. Drain and dry on paper toweling.

2. Place sprouts in colander. Rinse under cold running water. Drain and dry on paper toweling.

3. Combine snow peas and sprouts and tomato in medium bowl. Add only enough salad dressing to moisten. Toss gently to coat.

4. Arrange lettuce leaves on 4 individual salad plates. Cover with equal amounts of salad mixture. Sprinkle with almonds and serve.

YIELD: Serves 4

## SPICY STUFFED TOMATOES

4 ripe medium tomatoes
5 hard-cooked eggs
3 tablespoons dry-curd cottage cheese
  (no salt added)
3 tablespoons Lime Salad Dressing
  (page 162)
½ teaspoon smoked yeast (optional;
  available in health food stores)
2 tablespoons finely minced celery
6 dashes ground red (cayenne) pepper
1 teaspoon chili con carne seasoning
  (no salt or pepper added)
1 tablespoon minced fresh parsley
  Crisp lettuce leaves and watercress
  sprigs

1. Cut slice from stem end of each tomato. Scoop out pulp and coarsely chop. Reserve tomato shells.

2. Cut eggs in half. Discard all but 1 egg yolk. Place egg whites and 1 yolk in small bowl. Mash.

3. Add cottage cheese and salad dressing. Mash again. Stir in smoked yeast, celery, spices, parsley, and chopped tomato pulp. Stuff reserved tomato shells with mixture.

4. Serve on crisp lettuce leaves garnished with watercress sprigs.

YIELD: Serves 4

## WATERCRESS-MUSHROOM SALAD

1 small bunch crisp watercress
½ pound firm crunchy fresh mushrooms, washed, dried, trimmed, and thinly sliced
5 to 6 tablespoons All-Purpose Salad Dressing (page 161)

1. Wash watercress under cold running water. Dry on paper toweling. (Do not squeeze dry or all the flavor of the green will run out.) Break off and discard tough ends. Place in bowl. Add mushrooms.

2. Just before serving, add salad dressing, using just enough to moisten. Toss gently and serve.

YIELD: Serves 4

VARIATIONS:

1. Try with Creamy Green Sauce (page 167). Arrange watercress and mushrooms on individual salad plates. Spoon Creamy Green Sauce over salad (do not toss). You can be very liberal with this sauce because it's particularly low in fat and calories.

2. Serve salad with Low-Calorie Tomato Salad Dressing (page 161) using as much dressing as you like, or Lime Salad Dressing (page 162) using no more than 5 tablespoons dressing.

# DESSERTS

You'll never believe that desserts that are so good for you could taste so good. Here's a quartet of goodies for the ice cream, cookie, and cake lover in all of us—plus two more for those of us who long for sweets that are different. Enjoy all six as alternates to fresh fruit and canned pineapple packed in its own juice.

## CHUNKY PEACH ICE

¾ cup pineapple chunks packed in its own juice, including all but ¼ cup juice
⅔ cup evaporated skim milk
¼ cup buttermilk (no salt added)
¼ teaspoon ground cinnamon
1 tablespoon medium-dry sherry or Cognac
2 large ripe peaches, peeled and coarsely chopped

1. Combine first 5 ingredients in blender or food processor. Purée on high speed for 1 minute until smooth.
2. Pour into freezer tray that has been rinsed in cold water. Place tray directly on metal in freezer. Cover and freeze until almost firm (about 2 hours).
3. Beat with portable electric mixer in tray, or turn into food processor and process on/off 3 times. Spoon back into freezer tray. Fold in chopped peaches. Return tray, covered, to freezer. This time, do not place tray in direct contact with metal. Freeze for 1½ to 2 hours, stirring once midway. Fully ripened ice should be creamy and semisoft.

YIELD: Serves 6

VARIATION: One-third cup sweet fresh blueberries may be substituted for 1 peach. The combination is delicious.

NOTE: Ices will harden when left in freezer overnight. To serve, remove from freezer and place in refrigerator for 1 hour. Remove from refrigerator and let stand at room temperature for 30 minutes, or until softened. The lower the temperature of the freezer, the longer the softening time.

## MOIST APPLE CAKE

1½ cups whole-wheat flour
¼ cup unbleached flour
3 teaspoons low-sodium baking powder
1 teaspoon ground cinnamon
½ teaspoon ground ginger
¼ cup toasted wheat germ (no sugar added)
½ cup date sugar (date powder)
2 eggs (use 1 yolk and 2 whites)
½ cup evaporated skim milk
¼ cup unsweetened pineapple juice
2 tablespoons each corn oil and sweet (unsalted) 100 percent corn oil margarine at room temperature, plus ¼ teaspoon margarine for pan
1 teaspoon pure vanilla extract
1 teaspoon grated orange rind, preferably from navel orange
3 cups peeled and coarsely chopped tart apples (about 3 apples)

1. Sift flours, baking powder, and spices into bowl. Stir in wheat germ and date sugar. Set aside.

2. In large bowl, beat eggs, milk, and juice with whisk until blended. Combine oil and 2 tablespoons margarine and whisk into mixture. Stir in vanilla and orange rind.

3. Add dry ingredients to egg mixture, ½ cup at a time, stirring with wooden spoon after each addition.

4. Fold in apples. (Mixture will be thick.) Spoon and spread into lightly margarine-greased 9-inch square baking pan. Bake in preheated 350°F oven for 50 to 55 minutes. Cake is done when it moves away from sides of pan and is lightly browned. Place pan on rack and let cool. Cut into 12 serving pieces and serve.

YIELD: 12 squares

VARIATION: In step 4, fold in ⅓ cup loosely packed raisins.

NOTE: Eat just *one* square for dessert. Freeze the balance. Reheat in aluminum foil for another day's treat.

## STEWED MANGOES

¼ cup apple juice (no sugar added)
1 tablespoon honey (optional)
1 tablespoon Cognac
⅛ teaspoon freshly grated nutmeg
½ teaspoon ground cinnamon
2½ cups ripe peeled and sliced mangoes
(about 2 medium mangoes)

1. Combine first 5 ingredients in small enameled saucepan. Bring to boil. Add mangoes. Bring to simmering point. Partially cover and simmer for 2 minutes (see note below). Remove from heat. Let cool, uncovered, in cooking juices. Transfer to jar and chill.

2. Serve in decorative individual dessert dishes *au naturel,* or with Whipped Creamy Topping (page 166).

YIELD: Serves 4

NOTES:

1. Cooking time will vary depending upon ripeness of fruit.

2. This dish can substitute for breakfast fruit.

## PLUM CAKE

### For the cake:

2  egg whites
⅛ teaspoon cream of tartar
1  egg yolk
1  tablespoon honey
2  tablespoons each corn oil and sweet (unsalted) 100 percent corn oil margarine, plus ½ teaspoon margarine for baking pan
2  tablespoons dry-curd cottage cheese (no salt added)
1  teaspoon grated orange rind, preferably from navel orange
1  teaspoon pure vanilla extract
½ cup whole-wheat flour
1  cup unbleached flour
4  teaspoons low-sodium baking powder (available in health food stores)
½ teaspoon ground cinnamon
¼ cup each orange juice (no sugar added) and evaporated skim milk
1¼ pounds ripe sweet purple plums (about 18 plums) washed, pitted, each plum cut into thirds

### For the topping:

2  tablespoons each unbleached flour and date sugar (date powder)
2  teaspoons sweet (unsalted) 100 percent corn oil margarine, softened
½ teaspoon ground cinnamon
¼ teaspoon ground allspice

1. Place egg whites in mixing bowl. Beat with cream of tartar until stiff but not dry. Set aside.
2. In another bowl, beat egg yolk, honey, oil, 2 tablespoons margarine, cottage cheese, orange rind, and vanilla extract with wire whisk until light and well blended.
3. Sift together flours, baking powder, and cinnamon. Combine orange juice and milk. Add sifted dry mixture to egg yolk mixture alternately with milk mixture. Fold in beaten egg whites. (Do not overfold.)
4. Lightly grease a 9-inch square baking pan with margarine. Spread batter evenly across pan. Arrange plums side by side, cut edges down, on top of batter in a neat pattern.
5. Combine all ingredients for topping in small bowl. Blend with spoon and then with fingers to make a crumbly texture. Sprinkle over plums.
6. Bake in preheated 350°F oven for 50 to 55 minutes. Insert toothpick between plums. Cake is done when toothpick comes out dry. Place pan on rack. Let cool for 10 minutes. Cut into 12 to 16 serving pieces. Serve warm or at room temperature.

YIELD: 12 to 16 portions

NOTE: This cake freezes magnificently. Wrap each portion in waxed paper, then place in paper bag. Place paper bag in plastic bag. Seal tightly and freeze. To serve, unwrap; lay on baking sheet. Cover loosely with aluminum foil, and bake in preheated 350°F oven for about 12 minutes, or until cake is heated through. Serve warm.

## TASTY MUNCHIN' COOKIES

1⅓ cup unbleached flour
¼ cup whole-wheat flour
⅓ cup date sugar (date powder)
½ cup crumbled spoon-size shredded
   wheat
2 teaspoons low-sodium baking powder (available in health food stores)
1½ teaspoons ground cinnamon
1 teaspoon each anise seed, crushed,
   and ground coriander
1 tablespoon grated orange rind, preferably from navel orange
2 tablespoons sweet (unsalted) 100
   percent corn oil margarine, plus ½
   teaspoon for cookie sheets
1 tablespoon corn oil
1 egg
2 tablespoons evaporated skim milk
¾ cup buttermilk (no salt added)
1 teaspoon pure vanilla extract

1. Combine first 8 listed ingredients in large mixing bowl. Stir to
blend.
2. In another bowl, beat 2 tablespoons margarine and the oil until
blended. Add egg and evaporated milk.
Beat until blended.
3. Add liquid mixture to dry mixture and beat until flours are moistened.
With mixing machine on, gradually add
buttermilk and vanilla. (Finished batter
will be thick.)
4. Drop by spoonfuls onto lightly
margarine-greased cookie sheets, flattening each cookie with moistened spoon.
Bake in preheated 400°F oven for 16 to
18 minutes, until browned on bottom
and lightly brown on top. Let cool thoroughly on rack before serving.

YIELD: 36 cookies

VARIATION: Add ⅓ cup raisins to batter
during step 3.

NOTE: Cookies may be crisped up next
day if necessary by baking for 5 minutes
in preheated 400°F oven.

## APRICOT BREAD

½ cup chopped dried unsulphured apricots

¾ cup apple juice (no sugar added)

1¼ cups unbleached flour

½ cup whole-wheat flour

3 teaspoons low-sodium baking powder (available in health food stores)

1 teaspoon ground cinnamon

¼ teaspoon ground allspice

¼ cup date sugar (date powder)

1 tablespoon toasted wheat germ (no sugar added)

2 tablespoons sweet (unsalted) 100 percent corn oil margarine, plus ¼ teaspoon for baking pan

1 tablespoon corn oil

1 egg

2 tablespoons honey (optional)

⅔ cup evaporated skim milk

1 teaspoon grated orange rind, preferably from navel orange

1 tablespoon Cognac

1. Place apricots in small bowl. Bring apple juice to boiling point. Pour over apricots. Stir to separate. Let stand while batter is being prepared.

2. Sift flours, baking powder, and spices into another bowl. Stir in date sugar and wheat germ. Set aside.

3. Whisk margarine with corn oil in large mixing bowl. Add egg and honey, whisking until smooth. Add softened apricots with apple juice from step 1. Then add flour mixture alternately with milk, stirring with wooden spoon after each addition.

4. Stir in orange rind and Cognac. Batter will be thick. Spoon into lightly margarine-greased loaf pan (7⅜ × 3⅝ × 2¼ inches). Bake in preheated 350°F oven for 45 to 50 minutes. Test for doneness: toothpick inserted into center of cake should come out dry.

5. Place pan on rack for 5 minutes. Loosen around sides of pan with blunt knife. Remove loaf from pan. Place on rack and let cool for at least 1 hour before slicing. Delicious served slightly warm or at room temperature.

YIELD: 15 slices

VARIATION: If you don't have Cognac on your shelf, you may substitute 1 teaspoon pure vanilla extract; and in step 1, add 1 teaspoon fresh lemon juice.

NOTE: This dish doubles as a breakfast stand-in for cereal and other carbohydrate food.

# 3

# WHAT'S YOUR PROBLEM ON COOKING FOR BETTER HEALTH?

***Do I have to go to a special cooking school to learn how to cook for better health?***

Oh, no! You can follow my recipes even if you've never cooked before. The instructions are so explicit that you'll think I'm standing beside you, giving you personal instruction.

I give you the details that spell the difference between a so-so dish and a delight. I don't generalize, as many cookbooks do—like, "Cook until brown." I *specify*, "Sauté over medium heat until lightly browned (about 2 minutes)." Nothing is left to chance.

***I have a tiny kitchen. I hope I don't need a lot of equipment to cook your way.***

You don't. The following utensils (some or all of which you may have already) will get you started at once:

- Nonstick skillet
- 1-quart saucepan
- Chopping board
- Measuring cups and measuring spoons
- Sharp knives
- Spatula
- Wire whisk
- Broiling pan with rack (it doubles as a roasting pan)
- Bowls of several sizes

After your initial successes, you'll become so excited you'll want to try your hand at cooking recipes using—

- Iron skillet
- Muffin pans
- Cookie sheets
- Loaf pans
- Grater
- Colander
- Food processor

When you're ready to cook *anything*, you'll find all the equipment you need listed in *The Dieter's Gourmet Cookbook.*

***How many kinds of knives do I need?***

To start with, all you need is three knives: a serrated knife for bread and vegetables; a sharp-edged 8-inch all-purpose knife for chopping and cutting vegetables, fish, poultry, and meat; and a small paring knife. You'll also find a swivel-bladed peeler indispensable for peeling potatoes, zucchini, and fruit.

***My problem is keeping a neat counter and sink when paring and trimming vegetables. I'd appreciate your suggestions.***

Place ingredients next to each other, and a sheet of wax paper close to them.

Drop wastes on it. When paring and trimming are completed, fold wax paper over wastes and discard. Quick and easy!

### I know frying is bad for me. Isn't sautéing the same as frying?

Frying means cooking in a great deal of oil, and that *is* bad for you because a lot of the oil is absorbed by the food. Excess fat (oil is liquid fat) is a health hazard and an appetite stimulant. Sautéing means cooking in a small amount of oil. You can't survive without *any* fat, and the small amount of oil helps you meet your body's needs. It's okay to sauté.

### Must I always use a nonstick skillet?

Almost always. With a nonstick skillet you can cook with a minimum amount of fat (oil) or none at all. When I require more intense heat than I can get with a nonstick skillet, I switch to an iron skillet. For instructions on "seasoning" an iron skillet, see Note page 130.

### What's the best way to skim off fat from soups and stocks?

Prepare the day before you expect to use. Pour into a glass container, cover tightly, and refrigerate. The fat will rise to the top and freeze into a solid layer. When ready to use, cut it away.

Here are three less efficient but faster ways to get rid of the fat:

1. Let liquid stand for 30 minutes, then blot surface with paper toweling.

2. Let liquid cool, then add a handful of ice cubes. Retrieve immediately with slotted spoon. The fat will form solid layers along the sides of the cubes.

3. Use a skimming utensil as directed.

### You crush dried herb leaves. Wouldn't it be easier to buy dried herb leaves that are already ground?

Yes, if they tasted as good. The flavors of dried herbs peak immediately after crushing. Also, there are some dried herbs that are available only in the leaf form—tarragon and chervil, for example. But if you can get *fresh* herbs, forget about the dried variety, leafed or crushed.

### What's the best way to chop fresh herbs?

Chop small amounts by hand, large amounts in a food processor. Take care that herbs are bone dry before processing or you'll get a watery end-product.

### I bought what I thought was parsley. It turned out to be dandelion leaves. How can I prevent making that mistake again?

Lots of people make that mistake. Flat (Italian) parsley and dandelion leaves are look-alikes at first glance. When in doubt, taste. I use curly or flat parsley for mincing, and curly parsley for garnish.

### I understand garlic has been called a wonder herb for its health-promoting properties. But when I eat garlic I get indigestion and bad breath. What shall I do?

Prepare garlic the right way and you'll be delighted, not distressed. Start by throwing away your garlic press. Never, never, never crush garlic. Mince it. Then sauté in a small amount of oil in a nonstick skillet. My recipes calling for garlic generally include minced fresh parsley as well. It's a natural breath freshener.

### I sometimes have difficulty finding salt-free buttermilk. Can I use plain low-fat yogurt instead?

Yes, but don't expect exactly the same results. Thin down the yogurt to the consistency of buttermilk with low-fat or no-fat milk.

### I've been told not to have alcohol. You use vermouth in some of your recipes. Is there a substitute?

You don't need one. The alcoholic content of the wine is completely dissipated during cooking. All that remains are the lovely flavors. Double-check with your physician.

*How can I beat egg whites until they're stiff? I don't seem to have much luck.*
Use a large-whisked electric beater or a copper bowl and a large whisk. Egg whites must be at room temperature, and contain not a smidgeon of yolk.

*You use natural sweeteners. Can I substitute artificial sweeteners?*
No. Artificial sweeteners distort natural flavors and impart that diet-y taste. Natural sweeteners—fruits, fruit juices, sweet herbs and spices—help make dishes taste the way you've always liked them.

*I just can't stand store-bought bread, but I don't have the patience to follow most bread recipes—they're so complicated.*
I know exactly what your problem is. That's why I've worked so hard to make my bread recipes simple and easy to follow. You'll not only get a crackling, delicious loaf the first time and every time, you'll also make a marvelous discovery: Breadmaking is one of the most exciting and satisfying of life's experiences.

*I love to make bread. But sometimes the dough just doesn't rise very high. What do I do wrong?*
One of two things. The water you add may not be hot enough (110° to 115° F.) to activate the yeast; or it may be too hot, and it kills some of the yeast.

There's also the possibility that you did nothing wrong; some of the yeast may have been dead to start with. That can happen even though you use it long before the expiration date stamped on the package.

It's a good idea to proof your yeast before adding to flour. To a cup con-

taining ¼ cup warm water (110° to 115° F) and ½ teaspoon honey (optional) add the amount of yeast called for in the recipe. Stir to dissolve, then let stand for 10 minutes. If the mixture thickens and puffs up, the yeast is fine.

*Can I substitute canned or frozen fruits and vegetables for fresh ones?*
No to regular canned vegetables because of the high salt content. (One cup of fresh peas has two milligrams of sodium; one cup canned peas, 401.) No to regular canned fruits because of their high sugar content. (There's less than 1 percent sucrose in a pound of fresh peaches; about 46 percent in a pound of canned peaches.) Dietetic canned foods are usually tasteless. Some exceptions: Low-sodium tomatoes, tomato paste, and tomato purée; tuna and salmon packed in water (not broth), no salt added; and pineapple packed in its own juice.

Frozen foods are acceptable when no sugar or salt is added. Be wary of frozen fish fillets; they may be treated with brine before freezing. And stay away from frozen lima beans. (One cup of fresh lima beans is virtually sodium free; one cup of frozen lima beans contains 232 milligrams of sodium.)

*I'm told if I specifically prepare foods for freezing I should slightly undercook. Is that correct?*
Yes. Then when you reheat, you avoid overcooking.

*I understand that overcooking destroys nutrients. Is that true?*
Yes. Nutritive values are diminished by 50 percent.

*What's the best way to retain the taste of freshly cooked foods when I freeze them?*
Cool food to room temperature immediately after cooking. To freeze stocks,

soups, vegetables, meats, or poultry in a sauce, fill plastic pouches or freezing containers and seal tightly. To freeze cooked meat or poultry without a sauce (don't freeze cooked fish) wrap tightly in waxed paper, then in aluminum foil, and freeze. When reheating, do not overcook. You'll be delighted with the natural flavor and texture of the food.

### Can I freeze raw or cooked stuffed poultry?
No, if it's homemade. The stuffing can go bad. It's wise to freeze the raw bird, then stuff when it's ready for the oven. Or cook the bird and stuffing, and freeze each separately. Commercial stuffed poultry usually contains additives that retard spoilage during freezing. Read the labels.

### What other approved foods on your diet shouldn't I freeze?
Low-fat milk; buttermilk; low-fat yogurt; eggs in a shell; hard-cooked eggs; raw potatoes; Chinese cabbage; dill (but you can freeze other herbs; they'll discolor, but their flavors will be virtually unaffected); potato salad and stews made with potatoes (but you can freeze baked and mashed potatoes); yeast dough; raw vegetables (chopped, grated, or sliced); pie crusts with fillings (but you can freeze each separately); meringues; seasoned meats and poultry; and cooked fish.

### Is there any way I can freeze eggs?
Yes. Remove from shell, cover, and place in an ice cube tray.

### Can I freeze pasta, rice, and cooked vegetables?
Yes, if they're a little underdone. But why would you want to when they cook so easily and rapidly? Frozen pasta, be warned, tends to stick together and lose flavor.

# HOW TO GET PERSONAL ANSWERS TO YOUR SPECIFIC QUESTIONS

Just write me care of my publisher:

Francine Prince
Cornerstone Library
Division of Simon and Schuster
1230 Avenue of the Americas
New York, NY 10020

I'll respond as soon as I can. Please enclose a stamped, self-addressed envelope.

# INDEX
# OF RECIPES

# General Index

aerobics, 87
age:
    ideal weight and, 34
    SDAs and, 79–81
    vitamin supplements and, 30, 31, 63
aging, exercise and, 86
Agriculture Department, U.S., 25, 78, 82, 92, 94
Air Force, U.S., exercises for, 87
airliners, dieting in, 60
alcohol, 69, 75
    substitutes for, 196–97
    vitamins and, 25, 31
allergies, food, 73
American restaurants, 60
amphetamines, 24
anemia, 17, 97
appestat, 21–23, 62, 75
    of compulsive eaters, 26–27
    defined, 21
    high setting of, 22–23, 26, 34, 36–37, 62, 73
    normal setting of, 21–22, 23, 26, 27, 33, 34, 37, 82, 97
Archer, Morton, 19
artery blockage, 19, 74
arthritis, 86
artificial sweeteners, 197
Atkins, Robert C., 62
Atkins Diet, 17
avocados, fats in, 74

bad breath, 17, 77
baking bread, 197
Baumgartner, Leona, 15–16
Beckwith, Patricia, 88
behavioral training, diets and, 76–77
Benowicz, Robert J., 24–25, 94
benzocaine, 24
beverages:
    guilt-free, 47
    Thin-for-Life, 66, 68
    see also alcohol
Beverly Hills Diet, The, 17

bicycles, exercise, 87
blood pressure, 19, 24, 81
    exercise and, 86
    salt and, 92, 93
Blumenfeld, Arthur, 16, 19
bone shrinkage, exercise as prevention against, 86
bread, 66, 74
    baking of, 197
    eating out and, 57
breakfast, 30
    Thin-for-Life, 66
Brody, Jane, 24
Bureau of Nutrition, New York City, 15–16
Burros, Marion, 93
butter, 39, 49, 58
buttermilk, salt-free, 196
B vitamins, 30, 31, 77, 78, 81, 97

cafeterias, dieting in, 60, 61
caffeine, 24, 25, 31
calcium, 31, 94, 97
calories, 15, 97
    appestat settings and, 21–23
    average consumption of, 82
    in condiments, 75
    empty, 74, 75, 93
    as measure of heat, 74–75
    vitamin requirements and, 78
cancer, 92, 93
canned foods, 63
    fresh foods vs., 197
carbohydrates, simple vs. complex, 93
cereals, 66
chain restaurants, dieting in, 61
*Chemical Nutrition* (Jolliffe), 18
chewing, 75, 77
chicken, skin of, 75
children, vitamins and, 31, 79–81
Chinese restaurants, 60
cholesterol, 27
    heart attacks and, 74, 92, 93
    safe intake of, 74

# THE DELICIOUS AND SENSIBLE DIET THAT CAN SAVE YOUR LIFE... OR THE LIFE OF SOMEONE YOU LOVE.

The sensational diet created by nationally acclaimed best-selling author Francine Prince.

## • NO SALT • NO SUGAR •
## • LOW  SATURATED FAT • LOW CHOLESTEROL

The THREE essential books for every health conscious American:

### THE DIETER'S GOURMET COOKBOOK

The original gourmet cookbook that can be used for any kind of restrictive diet. Indulge in over 200 delectable diet recipes that will excite even the most discerning palate.

### NEW GOURMET RECIPES FOR DIETERS

By popular demand, here are over 200 *new* and delicious recipes from around the world that anyone can create!

### DIET FOR LIFE

The complete dietary program that tells you how to help prevent and fight such degenerative diseases as high blood pressure, diabetes, hypoglycemia, atherosclerosis, strokes, and heart attacks. This is the first time Francine Prince's revolutionary principles have been assembled in a single program, in what could be one of the most valuable books you'll ever own. Includes 100 recipes.

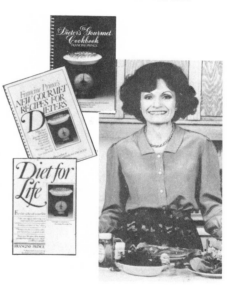

## • NO DRUGS • NO DISAGREEABLE THERAPIES
## • NO TASTELESS, ORDINARY DIET FOODS

Rather, the diet is so DELICIOUS and VARIED that it fights off the temptation to binge or stray.

Based on sound nutritional principles approved by:
American Medical Assoc.
American Heart Assoc.
Other leading medical authorities

YOU OWE IT TO YOURSELF AND THE PEOPLE YOU LOVE.